Postbiotics: Science, Technology and Applications

Authored by

Amin Abbasi

Department of Food Science and Technology
Faculty of Nutrition and Food Sciences
Nutrition Research Center
Tabriz University of Medical Sciences
Tabriz
Iran

Elham Sheykhsaran

Drug Applied Research Center
Department of Microbiology
Faculty of Medicine
Tabriz University of Medical Sciences
Tabriz
Iran

&

Hossein Samadi Kafil

Drug Applied Research Center
Department of Microbiology
Faculty of Medicine
Tabriz University of Medical Sciences
Tabriz
Iran

Postbiotics: Science, Technology and Applications

Authors: Amin Abbasi, Elham Sheykhsaran and Hossein Samadi Kafil

ISBN (Online): 978-1-68108-838-9

ISBN (Print): 978-1-68108-839-6

ISBN (Paperback): 978-1-68108-840-2

need for a court order if at any point you breach any terms of this License Agreement. In no event will any delay or failure by Bentham Science Publishers in enforcing your compliance with this License Agreement constitute a waiver of any of its rights.

3. You acknowledge that you have read this License Agreement, and agree to be bound by its terms and conditions. To the extent that any other terms and conditions presented on any website of Bentham Science Publishers conflict with, or are inconsistent with, the terms and conditions set out in this License Agreement, you acknowledge that the terms and conditions set out in this License Agreement shall prevail.

Bentham Science Publishers Ltd.
Executive Suite Y - 2
PO Box 7917, Saif Zone
Sharjah, U.A.E.
Email: subscriptions@benthamscience.net

BENTHAM SCIENCE

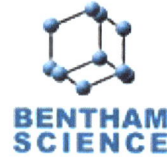

CONTENTS

PREFACE

Probiotics, prebiotics, and postbiotics are the main ingredients of functional foods that have recently become popular with researchers. Live probiotic cells and their derived postbiotics are frequently applying in commercial pharmaceutical and food-based products. The results of studies demonstrated that these bioactive elements could be linked with the host's cellular processes and metabolic pathways and possess a vital role in preserving and reestablishing host health. Despite the appropriate outcomes from the use of live probiotics, scientists have presented the postbiotic theory to find its precise mechanisms of action or optimize beneficial effects as well as to meet the requirements of customers to offer a safe product with a health claim. Currently, the scientific literature confirms that a large part of the molecular mechanism of probiotics is related to their derived postbiotics. These biomolecules, due to their unique pharmacokinetic properties, could be used, in their pure form and with high performance in veterinary, medical, and food practice to improve animal growth rate and health status, prevent and/or treat some acute/chronic diseases, and develop functional foods.

On the other hand, postbiotics with their unique features in terms of clinical, technological, and economic aspects can be applying as a promising approach (as potential alternative agents for probiotics and common antibiotics) in the food and drug industry for rising food safety and health effects as well as therapeutic targets. The fermentation process is the most natural production method of postbiotics, which enriches the fermented food matrices with these biomolecules. Nevertheless, postbiotics can be generated in a purer form and with high performance through several laboratory manners, which have the potential to be applied to an extensive range of food matrices to develop their nutritional values, storage stability, and health-promotion aims in customers. In the industry, manufacturers cannot easily add ingredients into the food matrix to produce functional food products that contain postbiotic compounds and, at the same time, have the desired quality and safety properties. Therefore it is indispensable that recognize the inherent characteristics of postbiotic compounds and select appropriate nanostructure carriers to design the best delivery system for the targeted delivery of postbiotics.

CONSENT FOR PUBLICATION

Not applicable.

CONFLICT OF INTEREST

The author declares no conflict of interest, financial or otherwise.

ACKNOWLEDGEMENTS

The authors would like to especially thank Dr. Hamideh Fathi Zavoshti for her helpful comments on the work.

Amin Abbasi
Department of Food Science and Technology
Faculty of Nutrition and Food Sciences
Tabriz University of Medical Sciences
Tabriz
Iran

Nutrition Research Center
Tabriz University of Medical Sciences
Tabriz
Iran

Elham Sheykhsaran
Drug Applied Research Center
Department of Microbiology
Faculty of Medicine
Tabriz University of Medical Sciences
Tabriz
Iran

&

Hossein Samadi Kafil
Drug Applied Research Center
Department of Microbiology
Faculty of Medicine
Tabriz University of Medical Sciences
Tabriz
Iran

ABOUT THE AUTHORS

Amin Abbasi was born in 1994 and is a Master of Science in Food Safety and Hygiene with significant contribution in science by publishing valuable articles in the well-known and top journals of food science and nutrition, and currently is working on probiotics and postbiotics in Food Science and Technology Department of Tabriz University of Medical Sciences.

Amin Abbasi
Department of Food Science and Technology
Faculty of Nutrition and Food Sciences
Tabriz University of Medical Sciences
Tabriz
Iran

Elham Sheykhsaran was born in 1989 and is a Ph.D. student of medical bacteriology with more than 25 publications in well-known journals of microbiology and currently is working on postbiotics in the Microbiology Department of Tabriz University of Medical Sciences.

Elham Sheykhsaran
Drug Applied Research Center
Department of Microbiology
Faculty of Medicine
Tabriz University of Medical Sciences
Tabriz
Iran

Dr. Kafil was born in 1983 and is an assistant professor of medical microbiology with more than 250 published papers and an h-index of 24. He finished his Ph.D. in medical microbiology, and his main topics of researches are clinical microbiology, immunology, and biotechnology. He has five patents on diagnosis methods. He currently works as the head of microbiology research in the Drug Applied Research Center and Imam Reza Hospital. Hossein is well-known for his antimicrobial approach and diagnostic innovations.

Hossein Samadi Kafil
Drug Applied Research Center
Department of Microbiology
Faculty of Medicine
Tabriz University of Medical Sciences
Tabriz
Iran

CHAPTER 1

Ecology of the Human Gastrointestinal Tract

Abstract: The digestive system has an explicit role in decomposing nutrients into energy and other necessary substances required by the body. The gastrointestinal tract contains a complex set of different microorganisms. It is considered the most dynamic and active organ in the body from a biological perspective. The environmental condition and daily diet are principal parameters that significantly influence the composition of gut microbiota. From birth to middle age, it undergoes significant changes. Several factors, such as maternal microbiota, birth status (natural, cesarean section), postpartum nutrition practices, microbial infections, overuse of antibiotics, diet (highly processed, low fiber), chronic diarrhea, and stress in life, have a significant effect on the gut microbiome. All of these factors lead to impaired bowel function and health. One of the most important strategies for overcoming dysbiosis conditions and establishing eubiosis conditions is the employment of foods containing probiotic, prebiotic, and postbiotic ingredients. Hence, this chapter provides a review of the concept and health-promoting issues regarding probiotics and prebiotics, with a focus on their biological role in the establishment of health.

Keywords: Dysbiosis, Eubiosis, Functional food, Gastrointestinal tract, Gut microbiota, Health, Postbiotic, Prebiotic, Probiotic.

INTRODUCTION

The digestive system has an explicit role in decomposing nutrients into energy and other necessary substances required by the body. In a person with a natural life span, about 60 tons of foodstuffs pass through the digestive tract. The gastrointestinal environment is a complex set of different microorganisms, which, from a biological perspective, are considered the most dynamic and active organs in the body [1, 2]. In addition to the central role of the gastrointestinal tract in the digestion and absorption of consumed nutrients, the complex metabolic activities in this episode have a well-known effect on human health. It is supposed that there are 10^{14} living microbes in the various part of the human body, even more than the number of cells in the human body, that is, approximately 10^{13} [3]. More than 400 different microbial species have been recognized in the samples of feces of a healthy individual, which in terms of microbial population is estimated to be about 10^{13} CFU/g. This number in the small intestine reaches 10^4-10^8 CFU/g, and in the stomach, only 10^1-10^2 CFU/g (Fig. **1**) [4].

Amin Abbasi, Elham Sheykhsaran & Hossein Samadi Kafil

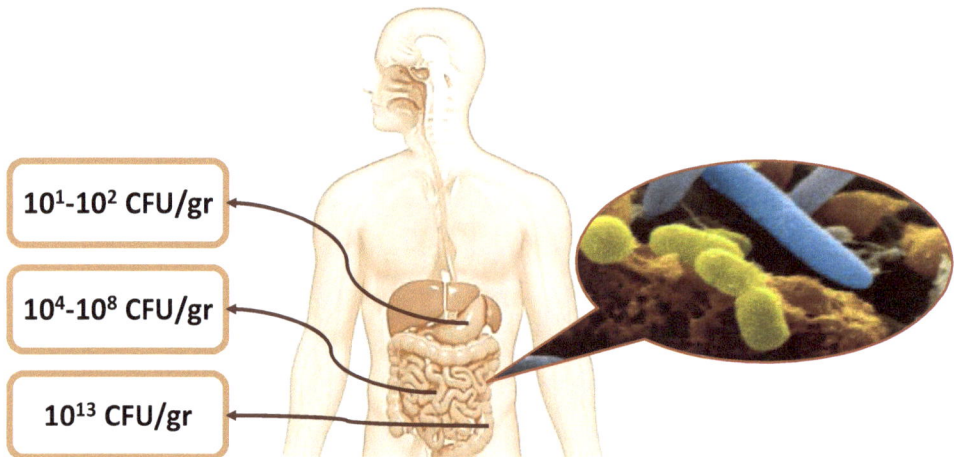

10^1-10^2 CFU/gr

10^4-10^8 CFU/gr

10^{13} CFU/gr

Fig. (1). Distribution of microbial species in different parts of the gastrointestinal tract.

The environmental condition and daily diet are principal parameters that significantly influence the composition of gut microbiota. From birth to middle age, it undergoes significant changes. During childbirth, the fetal gastrointestinal tract is free of any bacteria and sterile, but immediately after birth, replacement of the bacteria begins from the mother's genital tract in this episode [5]. Some factors such as sanitary conditions, type of delivery (normal-cesarean section), maternal microbial flora, nutrition, and other environmental factors potentially influence the composition of the gut microbial species [6]. During the first few days, the species *Coliform*, *Enterococcus*, *Clostridium*, *Lactobacillus*, and *Bifidobacterium* appear and form the dominant gut microbiota until the end of the first week. Therefore, in infants fed with breast milk, the bacterial population reaches 10^{10} CFU/gr of stool. It is a general rule that the type of feeding (breast or formula) significantly affects the composition of the microbial population in the baby's digestive tract [7, 8]. In the gastrointestinal tract of breast-fed infants, the levels of *Bifidobacterium* species are higher than those fed with formula, which in turn reduces the population of facultative anaerobic bacteria in this ecosystem. On the other hand, breast milk has less buffering power than formula and plays a significant role in intestinal acidification. This acidity act as a growth-inhibitor and inhibits the growth and development of *Clostridia* and *Bacteroides* sp, which in turn provides a specific platform for the growth of *bifidobacteria* (Table **1**) [9].

Besides, breast milk contains natural oligosaccharides, which are a stimulant for the growth of beneficial bacteria. So, it can be stated that breast milk contains thousands of bioactive compounds that boost the pediatric immune system and significantly affects the digestive tract ecosystem. When mothers decide to start the weaning process, *i.e.*, "mother-led weaning," the population and composition of gut microbes undergo noticeable changes. In this condition, the residents of *Bifidobacteria* spp. decrease, and the species of Bacteroides form the dominant intestinal flora [10]. The population and composition of adult gut microbiota are almost constant. Still, it can alter with increasing age so that significant changes in this composition (diminution in the quantity of *bifidobacteria* sp and an increase in pathogenic bacteria such as *Clostridium perfringens*) cause diarrhea in elderly individuals [11, 12]. In addition to age, other factors that can disrupt this microbial balance may include genetics, geographic location, weather, economic conditions, lifestyle, stress, chronic diseases, the overdose of medication, microbial corruption, and diet. Interestingly, any change in this microbial balance will allow for the dominance of pathogenic germs, which in turn may cause a variety of diseases (Fig. **2**).

Several factors such as maternal microbiota, birth status (natural, cesarean section), postpartum nutrition practices, microbial infections, overuse of antibiotics, diet (highly processed, low fiber), chronic diarrhea, and stress in life, have a significant effect on the gut microbiome that all of these factors lead to impaired bowel function and health [13]. One of the main side-effects is dysbiosis, a state in which microbial balance is disturbed, and pathogenic germs are created the dominant population in the gut environment. The use of antibiotics for a long time to treat chronic diseases such as diabetes, cystic fibrosis, tuberculosis, arthritis, cancer, *etc.*, is one of the most important causes of dysbiosis [14, 15]. "Eubiosis" is also a condition against dysbiosis, which refers to establishing a microbial balance in the gut ecosystem. In these conditions, *Bifidobacterium* and *Lactobacillus* species are predominant and possess health-promoting effects [16, 17]. One of the most important strategies for overcoming dysbiosis conditions and the establishment of eubiosis conditions is the use of foods containing probiotic, prebiotic, and postbiotic ingredients [18]. The application of probiotics and synbiotics in the food industry, with gut homeostasis promoting goal, have been blooming during the past decade. With the advances of science, the role of probiotics and symbiotic is more evident in the treatment of diseases. However, in some cases, probiotics or synbiotics do not exhibit the appropriate efficiency. In this regard, scientists investigate the activity and characteristics of soluble factors (postbiotics) derived from probiotics. So, discussing the definition of some terms, history, and their applications in the food industry seems to be necessary. We have heard this sentence repeatedly: there is a strong relationship between drinking milk and longevity. Metchnikoff's works and intentions were considering as the new phrase as probiotics. Probiotics are beneficial microbes to promote health. Nowadays, it is elucidated that, in the intestine, some beneficial microorganisms protect them against diseases. It is well explicates that gut microbiota has deficiencies to deal with pathogens. Hence, it is a necessity to get probiotics through the diet. Supplements containing probiotics repair these shortages.

Table 1. Distribution of microbial species in different parts of the gastrointestinal tract.

Microbial Species	Mouth	Stomach	Duodenum	Jejunum-ileum	Colon
Total count (number per g/ml)	10^8	10^1-10^2	10^1-10^3	10^3-10^6	10^{17}
Actinomyces spp	-	-	-	10^3-10^6	-
Bacteroides-Prevotella-Clostridium spp	-	10^1-10^2	10^1-10^3	10^4-10^7	10^9-10^{11}
Bifidobacterium spp	-	-	-	-	10^9-10^{10}
Clostridium spp	-	-	-	10^4-10^5	10^8-10^9
Coprococcus cutactus spp	-	-	-	-	10^7-10^8
Entrobacteriace spp	-	10^1-10^2	10^2-10^4	10^3-10^6	10^5-10^7
Enterococcus spp	-	-	-	10^2-10^4	10^3-10^6
Eubacterium spp	-	-	-	-	10^9-10^{11}
Fusobacterium spp	-	-	-	10^3-10^5	10^5-10^7
Lactobacillus spp	-	10^1-10^3	10^2-10^4	10^3-10^6	10^5-10^8
Metanobacteria	-	-	-	-	10^1-10^9
Peptostreptococcus spp	-	-	-	10^2-10^6	10^8-10^9
Proteus spp	-	-	-	-	10^3-10^6
Pseudomonas spp	-	-	-	-	10^3-10^6
Staphylococci	-	-	-	-	10^3
Streptococcus spp	-	10^1-10^3	-	10^3-10^8	10^7
Yeast spp	-	-	-	-	10^3

Psychological tensions ↑ Psychological tensions ↓

Microbial infections ↑ Microbial infections ↓

Taking antibiotics ↑ Taking antibiotics ↓

Highly processed foods ↑ Highly processed foods ↓

Birth status (cesarean) Birth status (normal)

Inappropriate diet Appropriate diet

Inappropriate living conditions Appropriate living conditions

Inappropriate economic conditions Appropriate economic conditions

Geographical location Geographical location

Dysbiosis **Eubiosis**

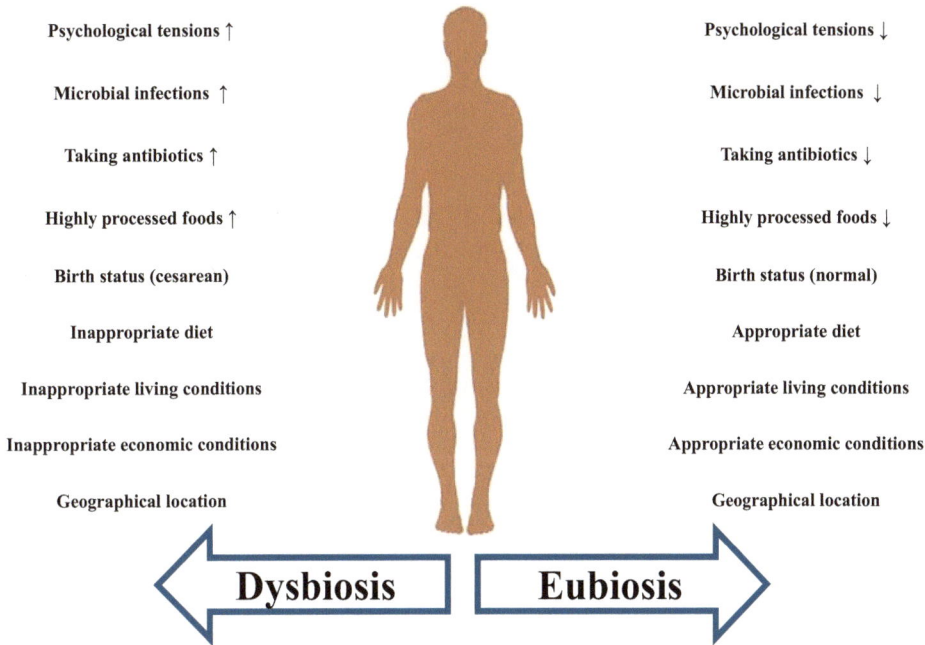

Fig. (2). Main factors in the establishment of Eubiosis and Dysbiosis in the gastrointestinal tract.

PROBIOTICS

Probiotic (probios, exact mean is life) are characterized as non-pathogenic microorganisms that exert beneficial effects on the host when consumed in sufficient quantities. FAO-WHO (Food and Agriculture Organization of the United Nations –World Health Organization) expert group consensus statement in 2001 confirms this definition of probiotics [19]. The fermentation process was first described by Louis Pasteur in the 1900s. Also, Metchnikoff (1907) explained the secret of longevity in the Bulgarian rural population in regular dairy product consumption. He considered the Lactobacilli as probiotics with positive effects on human health in particular gut regularity functions [20]. At the end of the First World War, major groups of children suffered from intestinal complications. Following the work of Metchnikoff, another researcher Isaac Carasso created in 1919 Danone in Barcelona where the production of yogurt from the Pasteur Institute took place utilizing ferments. Later, Rettger and Cheplin in 1921 demonstrated that *Lactobacillus acidophilus* implantation in the human gut could help fight diarrhea, constipation, and other intestinal complications. Meanwhile, in 1917 an *Escherichia coli* strain was isolated by Nissle (1918) which successfully treated acute cases of infectious gut complications like salmonellosis and shigellosis. This strain is a typical example of a non-lactic acid bacteria probiotic available in the market and sold as Mutaflor® (Ardeypharm GmbH, Germany). Nevertheless, probiotics history returns to 10000 years ago. In the Indian ancient culture, the consumption of milk was considered the main diet. Approximately 3200 BC, produced fermented milk by the Egyptians and also dairy products during the pharaonic period has referred to the usage of probiotics in ancient times.

The term '-biotics' is associated with the dietetic approaches, which can be applied to the gut microbiota direction towards a more beneficial state to host health. The 'biotic' term has a Greek root biotik-ós, meaning 'about life' and refers to the biological ecosystem including living organisms in a mutualistic relationship with their physical environment [21, 22]. *Lactobacillus, Bifidobacterium,* and *Streptococcus* genera have immunomodulatory ability and display positive functions. In children, probiotics play an essential role in treating some complications such as allergy, irritable bowel syndrome, and respiratory infections [23 - 25]. However, in immunocompromised cases, probiotics must be taken cautiously [18].

The principal part of the probiotic products includes a well-known and limited list of bacterial taxa that include mostly lactic acid bacteria (LAB) like the *Bifidobacterium* spp., and *Lactobacillus* spp. That has the potency to be generally regarded as safe (GRAS) [26]. The diversity of probiotics has always been increasing, *i.e.*, modern investigations lead to the recognition of the new races and species that include useful traits for humans. Also, probiotics have been divide into two scopes including general and provisional types in terms of efficiency. *Lactobacillus acidophilus* and *Bifidobacterium* are considered probiotics under any conditions. Other genera such as *Bacillus* and *Escherichia* in specific circumstances are placed in the probiotics category, for instance, in animals. Nevertheless, the selection criteria for probiotics are as follow;

- Be GRAS (Generally recognized as safe) and not toxic or pathogenic
- Preferably be a member of normal flora with human origin
- Resistance to pH, bile salts
- The ability of desirable attachment to epithelial cells
- High potential for proliferation and colonization
- Resistance to antibiotics, bacteriophages, and detrimental bacteria such as *Helicobacter pylori, Listeria monocytogenes, etc.* [27].

In addition to the above cases, cost-effectiveness is almost of importance in this regard. It has been evident that the gut microbiota can be affected by probiotics through the prohibition of pathogens by preventing their adhesion and colonization in the gut. Moreover, probiotics probably exert a critical role in the development of the immune system, synthesis of important nutrient components like vitamins, and improvement of the intestinal barrier integrity through the up-regulation of involved genes in tight junction signaling [28 - 30].

Beneficial Properties of Probiotics

Beneficial Properties of Probiotics Several investigations have been performed regarding the valuable benefits of probiotics on human health through animal studies or trials. Some of the properties are as follows:

- Anticancer activity [31].
- Prevention of allergic responses [32].
- Decreasing serum cholesterol [33].
- Stimulation of the immune system [34].
- Improvement of lactose malabsorption [35].
- Positive effects on gut microbiota [36].
- Improvement of the gut functions [37].
- Prevention of detrimental bacteria growth [38].

Probiotic and Gut Microbiota

For decades, the potential health benefits of probiotics have been an area of growing scientific interest. The positive benefits of probiotic supplements have been investigating in various diseases, including gastrointestinal and metabolic disorders where the outcomes of the studies have supported the potential application of probiotics as therapeutic agents [39 - 41].

Probiotics exert their health-promoting impact on the host by several possible mechanisms that entail: amelioration of intestinal barrier function by influencing the epithelium and mucus lining; manipulating intestinal microbial communities; producing antimicrobial elements; competitive relation with pathogenic germs; balancing luminal acidity, immune-modulation; and stimulating proliferation and differentiation of epithelial cells [42, 43].

Researches have attributed the beneficial effects of probiotic consumption to several health outcomes. A growing series of studies have highlighted the significant effects of probiotic consumption in particular health pathologies; moreover, there is still substantial evidence that supports the health-promoting effects of probiotics in healthy individuals [44]. Hou *et al.* found that *Firmicutes, Bacteroidetes, Proteobacteria, Actinobacteria,* and *Tenericutes* were the predominant phyla in the fecal microbiota of all healthy participants [43]. The prevalent indicator of the gut microbiota composition is the F/B ratio. The gut microbiota composition in healthy grown-ups and the discrepancies in their responses to the same probiotic intervention are considered principal factors in defining their roles in human health and wellbeing.

In recent centuries, the composition of the host gut microbiota has received much consideration as a significant risk factor for disease progression that has the potential to be manipulated through probiotic consumption. The findings of several studies indicated the relationship between some gut microbiota and metabolic diseases such as obesity, diabetes, and gastrointestinal diseases [44 - 46]. Besides, other gut microbiotas are necessarily involved in functional processes such as digestion of indigestible nutrients, and the production of vitamins and micronutrients [47]. Taken all together, the gut microbiota population and any alternations in its composition, are closely attributed to human health. Hence, the health-effects of probiotic consumption on gut microbiota could be exploited as a tool for the maintenance and promotion of host health.

Modulation of the Intestinal Microbiota by the Application of Probiotics

The concept of probiotics to the scientific community was introduced by Nobel laureate Elie Metchnikoff. He reported that the longevity of Bulgarians was related to the consumption of viable *Lactobacilli* contained fermented milk products [48]. The observation suggested that ingestion of certain microbes may exert a beneficial role in human health. Since then, probiotics as dietary supplements or functional foods had been widely exploited. The gut microbiome supports the function and integrity of the gastrointestinal tract, maintenance of immune homeostasis, and host energy metabolism [49]. Intestinal dysbiosis, an imbalance in microbial communities, leads to disrupted interactions between microbes and their host. The alternations of the microbiome composition and function may underlie susceptibility to various diseases [50]. Several lines of evidence have revealed the link between gut dysbiosis and chronic low-grade inflammation and metabolic disorders, which consequently lead to metabolic syndrome (*e.g.* obesity and diabetes), infections in the gastrointestinal tract, inflammatory bowel disease (IBD), and irritable bowel syndrome (IBS) [49, 51, 52].

Maintaining the richness and diversity balance of the intestinal microbiome is being achieved by treatment methods. Probiotics can represent positive functions in the gastrointestinal tract or increase the functionality of resident microbial communities. This characteristic of probiotics arises from competition for nutrients, secretion of growth substrates or inhibitors, and modulation of intestinal immunity. The findings of randomized controlled clinical trials supporting the positive effects of probiotics during the treatment of gastrointestinal diseases [42, 53 - 55].

Antimicrobial agents/metabolic compounds secreted by probiotics result in growth suppression of other microorganisms or competing for receptors and binding sites on the intestinal mucosa [56, 57]. It has been showing that *Lactobacillus* strains improve the integrity of the intestinal barrier, which subsequently can result in preservation of immune tolerance, reduction of bacterial translocation across the intestinal mucosa, and disease phenotypes such as gastrointestinal infections, IBS, and IBD [58]. Furthermore, probiotics can regulate gut immunity and the intestinal epithelial' responsiveness and immune cells to microorganisms in the intestinal lumen [59].

Several tools and methods have been applied to study the effects of probiotics on the composition, diversity, and function of the gut microbiota. The result of a clinical study indicates the diminished pain and flatulence in patients with IBS after receiving a 4-week rose-hip drink containing 5×10^7 CFU/ml of *L. plantarum* DSM 9843 daily [60]. The amelioration of the clinical symptoms was attributed to the attendance of *L. plantarum* and reduced amounts of *enterococci* in fecal specimens of patients. A more recent study regarding patients with diarrhea-dominant IBS (IBS-D) demonstrated symptomatic relief after administration of a probiotic mixture of *L. acidophilus, L. plantarum, L. rhamnosus, Bifidobacterium breve, B. lactis, B. longum,* and *Streptococcus thermophilus.* Remarkably, fecal microbiota analysis of the patients applying denaturing gradient gel electrophoresis (DGGE) revealed that in probiotics-treated patients the microbial composition was more stable than those of the placebo group [61]. Recent advancements in DNA sequencing and bioinformatics have opened new horizons in the field of the human microbiome and how various treatment methods can alter the composition and function of the microbial populations. Recently, using a high-throughput, culture-independent method, research conducted to analyze the fecal microbiota of 6-month old infants treated with supplements of *L. rhamnosus* (LGG) per day. Their findings illustrated the abundance of LGG and an increased evenness index in the fecal microbiota of these infants, which in turn suggests ecological stability [62]. In another study, the ability of probiotics in the alternation of gut microbiota was investigated using 16S rRNA metagenomic sequencing in *L. reuteri*-treated neonatal mouse model. Their results demonstrated a transitory augmentation in community evenness and diversity of the distal intestinal microbiome in *L. reuteri*-treated animals in comparison to the vehicle-treated animals [63]. The microbial population diversity is related to the increased ecological stability. So, probiotics can modify intestinal microbiota and stabilize microbial communities [64].

Further, probiotics may also modulate the global metabolic function of the intestinal microbiome. In gnotobiotic mice and monozygotic twins administration of fermented milk products containing several probiotic strains did not alter the composition of the intestinal bacterial population [65]. However, fecal meta-transcriptomic analysis in probiotics-treated animals revealed significant alternations in the expression of microbial enzymes (particularly enzymes of carbohydrate metabolism). Additionally, mass spectrometric analysis of urinary metabolites demonstrated abundant levels of several carbohydrate metabolites. To sum up, these observations proposed that probiotics may lead to the global metabolic function of the intestinal microbiome.

Modulation of Gut Microbiota-brain Axis by Probiotics

The gut and the brain are closely associated with 200-600 million neurons [66]. It has been evident that brain signals may affect the motor, sensory, and secretory modalities of the gastrointestinal tract, besides, the gut's visceral messages can alter brain function, though, and there is a reciprocal interaction between the gut and the brain [67, 68]. Since expanding evidence validated the indispensable role of gut microbiota in the gut-brain axis, the concept may be reconsidered as the gut microbiota-brain axis [69 - 72]. Nonetheless, the interaction pathways (possibly through neural, endocrine, and immune pathways) of gut microbiota (and/or metabolites produced by microbiota) and the brain are still far from being fully elucidated [73]. A growing body of evidence demonstrated that probiotics can modulate reciprocal interaction between gut microbiota and the brain and exert favorable impacts on brain activity and behavior. The safety aspects such as surviving in the gastrointestinal tract and non-pathogenicity with the human origin must be taken into account in probiotic strains used for human consumption [74].

Although the relationship between gut microbiota and mental disorders is complex, it is possible to improve the mentioned disorders through modulation of gut microbiota by probiotics consumption. For instance, Bercik *et al.* showed that *Bifidobacterium longum* results in normalized anxiety-like behavior induced by the noninvasive parasite *Trichuris muris* infection [74]; Bravo *et al.* illustrated that *Lactobacillus rhamnosus* (JB-1)-treated *Trichuris muris*-infected mice results in reduced anxiety- and depression-related behavior. Consumption of certain probiotics may affect brain activity in humans. Two-month administration of *Lactobacillus casei* strain Shirota in patients with chronic fatigue syndrome caused significant augmentation of both *Lactobacillus* and *Bifidobacterium* and a substantial decrease in anxiety symptoms in patients treated with the probiotic [74]. In another study oral administration of *L. helveticus* R0052 and B. longum R0175 ameliorated anxiety and depressive symptoms in healthy volunteers after 2 weeks of consumption, which was measured by the Hopkins Symptom Checklist (HSCL-90), the Hospital Anxiety and Depression Scale (HADS). Similarly, four-week administration of fermented milk product with probiotics (FMPP) (comprising *Bifidobacterium animalis* subsp. lactis, *Streptococcus thermophiles*,

Lactobacillus bulgaricus, and *Lactococcus lactis* subsp. lactis) to the healthy women, changed control central processing of emotion and sensation in the brain, including affective, viscerosensory, and somatosensory cortices [75].

Several studies tried to define probiotics' mechanisms of action that are involved in gut-brain axis signaling. Altered gut microbiota composition is related to brain anomalies. Probiotics can relatively or completely balance the dysbiosis of the microbiota induced by some brain diseases. Vagus nerve-mediated, immune response-mediated, and metabolite-mediated pathways are among different pathways involved in the modulation of the gut microbiota-brain axis. Developing novel microbial-based therapeutic approaches for brain diseases relies on a deeper understanding of gut bacteria communication and their hosts.

Dietary supplementation may probably alter the composition of the gut microbiota in infants and adults. Probiotics are considered as preventive and therapeutic measures, which may lead to the maintenance of the healthy gut microbiome composition and function. Identification of new indigenous microbial species and tools as a result of human microbiome studies can positively modify the gut microbial populations. Well-designed experiments in applicable experimental models (*in vitro* or *in vivo*) may increase understandings of the biology and potential manipulation of the microbiome in the human host. Novel probiotic strains and medicinal components produced by the microbiome may be exploited as future strategies to promote health and prevent/treat different diseases.

PREBIOTICS

For two recent decades, researchers Professor Roberfroid, Gibson introduced the concept of prebiotics. This term has become an interesting topic in science in different fields, in particular biomedical and nutrition. A majority group of non-digestible oligosaccharides (NDOs) is consists of 3–10 sugar moieties including glycosidic bonds in the beta-configuration, therefore, rendering the endogenous enzymes of animals including fish-resistant and hydrolysis are implemented to the alpha glycosidic linkage recognition as a typical in starch [76]. Oligosaccharides prebiotic can provide the essential energy for selecting responsible bacterial species to the product of short-chain organic acids. Indeed, metabolic cross-feeding is a process whereby metabolites from one bacterial species are the source of energy to other bacteria with the resulting short-chain fatty acids (SCFAs) production, primarily lactic, propionate, acetate, and butyrate. The functional properties of prebiotics presumably induce production of SCFA leads to blood lipid modulation, energy sources resulting in intestinal cell proliferation, GI/systemic immunomodulation, and improved intestinal barrier function improvement. Decreasing pH aids general nutritional support and absorption of minerals. The synergistic promotion of symbiotic and commensal microorganisms provides the competitive exclusion of pathogens, decreasing toxic microbial metabolites, and preventing intestinal inflammation [77]. The SCFAs have a crucial role in the growth and intestinal tissue physiology and systemic metabolism in animals and humans to produce a large proportion of colonocytes' energy requirements. Limited knowledge for the fish is available however, it has been demonstrated that enterocytes of fish can absorb SCFAs. Acetate acts as a primary fuel for the heart, brain, and skeletal muscle. Propionate stimulates the crypt cells of the absorptive epithelium in mammals. Also, it has been revealed that propionate can reduce the output of hepatic glucose and modulate biosynthesis cholesterol. Butyrate, as the most common SCFAs is produced by gut microbiota and accounts for the oxygen requirements for the intestinal microorganisms in fish. The fatty acid presumably up-regulates glutathione S-transferase and expression of catalase in the distal intestine. The latter is crucial animal enzymes that belong to the primary antioxidant enzyme system and help suppress free radical generation and oxidative stress. Also, butyrate is correlating with the osmoregulation processes of the intestine and sodium absorption [18, 78].

Beneficial Properties of Prebiotics

The main health-promoting effects of prebiotics on human health include; a) reducing cancer risk, b) balancing cholesterol levels, c) increasing minerals' absorption, d) promoting hormonal balance, e) regulating lipid metabolism, f) lowering the risk of cardiovascular disease, g) decreasing acute gastroenteritis, h) and lowering autoimmune reactions. Recently, a growing interest in prebiotics has been conducted, which selectively enhances useful components of the intestine microbiota. Their use is directing towards favoring beneficial compounds within the gut microbial milieu like the lactobacilli and bifidobacteria. They are distinct from most dietary fibers such as cellulose, xylan, and pectin. These components are not selectively metabolized by intestine microbiota. Contrary to probiotics, prebiotics can be added to different foods such as baked or cooked since they lack the survivability issues related to probiotics [79]. The fructan such as oligofructose, inulin, and no sugar are present market leaders to prebiotics across the globe. The majority of fructan is either synthesized from sucrose or commercially prepared inulin-rich plant sources like the chicory root (Cichorium intybus). Nevertheless, several alternative sources of inulin, including burdock (Arctium lappa) Jerusalem artichoke (JA) (Helianthus tuberosusand) are currently being commercialized, and there is increasing scientific supportive literature of their equivalence to chicory-derived inulin. These prebiotics as emerging candidates probably finds their way into the world market. Nevertheless, there is a need to approve their efficiency utilizing reliable methodologies in various trials and formulations.

THE CONSUMPTION OF FUNCTIONAL FOODS AND THE ESTABLISHMENT OF GASTROINTESTINAL HEALTH

The results of studies in recent decades have highlighted the positive role of food in the hosts' health and quality of life. In this respect, the primary function of diet, as a source of energy, has changed to its biological role in preventing various types of diseases and creating a variety of health-promoting effects on the host (human and/or animal). Antimicrobial, antioxidant, immunomodulation, and anti-cancer activities are well-known examples of their biological roles. It is noteworthy that such activities are closely related to the presence of various compounds with bioactive properties in the matrix of various (dairy and non-dairy) foods. Therefore, many efforts have been made to develop functional foods, a specific type of foods that in addition to their basic nutritional value and primary role in energy supplying have particular health effects on the host [80]. In general, these foods may promote general body circumstances (*e.g.* probiotics), diminish the risk of certain diseases (*e.g.* cholesterol-lowering products), and potentially be implicated in the prevention and treatment of various diseases. Through the years, these foods have started as foods enriched with vitamins and/or minerals (Food, Vitamin C, Vitamin E, Folic Acid, Zinc, Iron, and Calcium) and have grown into foods that promote healthy nutrition and prevent various diseases, containing micronutrients such as omega-3 fatty acids, phytosterols and soluble fibers [81].

Today, along with increasing awareness and acceptance of consumers, the consumption of functional foods in the world, especially Europe, America, and Japan, has spread dramatically. The results of clinical studies indicate a significant relationship between lifestyle (especially diet), a variety of diseases, and consumer health status. In this regard in 1990, functional foods were first marketed in Japan to prevent chronic diseases such as diabetes, hypertension, cancer as well as reducing health care costs [82]. In recent years, along with increasing awareness and reporting of beneficial effects of functional foods on health status, scientific communities, manufacturers, and consumers have shown great interest in these groups of foods. So that the production and consumption of functional foods in developed countries such as Europe, America, and Japan have significant progress. However, some countries lack it for several scientific and economic reasons. Japan is one of the countries with a piece of good knowledge about functional foods, and it is usually considering one of the leading countries in the formulation, production, consumption, and setting of relevant standards in this field [83]. Various factors such as high costs of treatments, un-favorable side effects of some treatment (in chronic diseases like cancer), the importance of prevention before treatment, consumer desire to consume a variety of foods with health-promoting benefits and ultimately improve the quality of life are the important reasons for the growing demand for functional foods [84]. In Europe, probiotics and prebiotic foods account for 60 percent of the market for functional foods, while in the US this is slightly lower. In Japan, 270 types of probiotic and prebiotic functional food products are formulated and manufactured, of which more than 46 are relating to protein and peptide compounds [85]. On the other hand, investigations on postbiotic compounds demonstrated higher stability of these compounds during the production process, storage (with a shelf-life of more than five years in foods and beverages), and the digestive tract conditions [86]. Consequently, due to the favorable characteristics of postbiotics in terms of safety, stability, pharmacokinetics, standardization, and transportation, they can utilize in a wide range of functional foods (fermented and/ or non-fermented) to enhance their nutritional value, shelf-life, and health-promotion goals for consumers [87].

CHAPTER 2

Obstacles and Challenges in the Use of Probiotics

Abstract: Probiotics are helpful microorganisms that are resistant to biliary, gastric, and pancreatic secretions and can attach to the epithelial cells and colonize the surface of the intestinal cells. These capabilities are the main mechanisms of probiotics that allow them the adaptation to gut conditions. Probiotic cells attach to the intestinal cells and inhibit the attachment of enteric pathogenic germs to the intestinal mucosa by producing growth-inhibitory elements such as short-chain fatty acids, bacteriocin, and toxic oxygen metabolites. Attaching to the mucosal layer is essential for their functions, but it can increase the possibility of translocation and pathogenicity. On the other hand, there are also concerns about the possible transmission of antimicrobial resistance properties from probiotic strains to pathogenic bacteria in the gut environment. Consequently, the use of probiotics is entirely safe only in healthy people, and also it should be used with caution in children, the elderly, pregnant women, and immunocompromised patients. In recent years, scientists take a new approach to using probiotics in a non-viable form (currently known as postbiotics) to overcome the technological, economic, and clinical problems regarding the application of live probiotics. Hence, this chapter provides an overview of the nutritional and clinical concerns caused by probiotic intake in vulnerable patients, with emphasis on the application of a non-viable form of probiotics as a promising alternative.

Keywords: Antibiotic-resistance genes, Biogenic amines, D-lactic acid, Functional foods, Postbiotic, Probiotic.

Probiotics are beneficial microorganisms that are resistant to biliary, gastric, and pancreatic secretions and can attach to the epithelial cells and colonize the surface of the intestinal cells [88, 89]. These probiotic abilities are the main mechanisms that allow them to adapt to gut conditions [90]. Many researchers believe that probiotics should stay alive in the gut environment and exert their beneficial effects by adhering to the gut epithelium [91]. Most probiotics belong to *Bifidobacterium* and *Lactobacillus* species [92]. Probiotics can be used as dietary supplements or therapeutic agents [93]. Today, lactic acid-producing bacteria have become fundamental microorganisms for producing fermented foods such as yogurt, cheese, and butter [94].

Amin Abbasi, Elham Sheykhsaran & Hossein Samadi Kafil

Probiotic bacteria are attached to the enterocytes and prevent the attachment of enteric pathogens to the intestinal mucosa by producing inhibitory substances such as bacteriocin, short-chain fatty acids, and toxic oxygen metabolites [95]. The attachment to the mucosal layer is essential for their functions, but it can increase the possibility of translocation and pathogenicity [96]. On the other hand, there are also concerns about the possible transmission of antimicrobial resistance properties from probiotic strains to pathogenic bacteria in the gut environment. Besides, the production of toxic metabolites such as biogenic amines and D-lactic acid is one of the main risks associated with the consumption of live forms of probiotics [97, 98]. Therefore, given the potential benefits of probiotic consumption, the application of these microorganisms has not always been of benefit. There are concerns about their use in clinical and industrial applications. Limited experiments have been conducted to control the quality of probiotic products and the potential risks associated with their use [99]. Although probiotic foods have many health benefits like other foods, they also have limitations that have received less attention. The limit of their use needs to be carefully studied and communicated to consumers.

NUTRITIONAL AND CLINICAL CONCERNS

Systemic Infections and Chronic Diseases

Case report studies have reported some cases of infections caused by probiotic intake in vulnerable patients. Most reports are about 12 cases of fungal infections caused by the presence of *Saccharomyces cerevisiae* and *Saccharomyces boulardii* in patients taking probiotics, and about eight cases of bacteremia have been reporting in association with *Lactobacillus* species [100]. Although the mortality has also been reported among others, in these cases, there was usually a pre-existing disease and not significantly related to probiotic-mediated infection. [88, 101, 102]. During the last ten years, many articles have been publishing to evaluate the safety profile of *Lactobacillus* based on tentative application to determine the pathogenicity of these microorganisms. There are thirteen species of *Streptococcus* in fermented foods [103] that are considered opportunistic pathogens and sometimes involved in human infections such as meningitis, endocarditis, bacteremia, and especially urinary tract infections [104]. The species of *Enterococcus* is resistant to many antibiotics, and some factors such as the presence of cell adhesion factors, production of cytolysin (hemolysin), presence of cell-surface proteins, extracellular superoxidase or zinc-containing metalloproteinase (gelatinase), contains M-like compounds, and leucine breakdown capability are involved in the pathogenicity of *Enterococcus faecalis*. These characteristics have led to doubts about the use of *Enterococci* as probiotics. Another undesirable feature of *Enterococci* is the presence of transmissible genes that encode resistance genes to antibiotics such as vancomycin [104, 105]. The most important concern about probiotics is the risk of infection [106]. According to the investigations, some diseases such as cancer, diabetes, and organ transplants (especially liver) significantly increase the chance of infection with *Lactobacillus* [107]. Table **2** illustrates some reports of infections caused by *Lactobacillus* and other probiotic species. Rautio *et al.* reported a liver infection in a 49-year-old woman with diabetes mellitus following the consumption of probiotic products containing *Lactobacillus rhamnosus* GG [108]. Table **3** lists *lactobacilli* and *bifidobacteria* commonly found in the intestine, as well as species associated with human infections [104].

Table 2. Bacterial infections associated with the use of probiotics in vulnerable individuals.

Probiotic Cell	Form of Sepsis	Age	Risk Factors	Method of Identification	References
Lactobacillus rhamnosus, 3×10^9 CFU/d	Endocarditis	67y	Mitral regurgitation, dental extraction	API 50 CH, pyrolysis mass spectrometry	[110]
LGG	Liver abscess	74 y	Diabetes mellitus	API 50 CH, PFGE of DNA restriction fragments	[108]
LGG	Bacteremia	3 mo	Prematurity, short gut syndrome	No confirmatory typing	[111]
LGG	Bacteremia	10 wk	Prematurity, inflamed intestine, short gut syndrome	PFGE of DNA restriction fragments	
LGG, 1/4 capsule/d	Bacteremia	11mo	Prematurity, gastrostomy, short-gut syndrome, CVC, parenteral nutrition, rotavirus diarrhea	rRNA sequencing	[112]
LGG, 10^{10} CFU/d	Endocarditis	4 mo	Cardiac surgery, antibiotic diarrhea	Repetitive element sequence-based PCR DNA fingerprinting	[113]
LGG, 10^{10} CFU/d	Bacteremia	6 y	Cerebral palsy, jejunostomy feeding, CVC, antibiotic-associated diarrhea	Repetitive element sequence-based PCR DNA fingerprinting	

Probiotic Cell	Form of Sepsis	Age	Risk Factors	Method of Identification	References
Bacillus subtilis, $8×10^9$ spores/d	Bacteremia	47 y	Not stated	Antibiotic susceptibility	[114]
Bacillus subtilis, $8×10^9$ spores/d	Bacteremia	25y	Not stated	Antibiotic susceptibility	
Bacillus subtilis, $8×10^9$ spores/d	Bacteremia	63 y	Neoplastic disease	Antibiotic susceptibility	
Bacillus subtilis, $8×10^9$ spores/d	Bacteremia	79 y	Not stated	Antibiotic susceptibility	
Bacillus subtilis, 10^9 spores/d	Bacteremia	73 y	Chronic lymphocytic leukemia	16S rRNA sequencing	[102, 115]

Table 3. *Lactobacilli* and *bifidobacteria* are commonly found in the human gut.

Microbial Species	Isolated From	
	Clinical Infections	Fermented Foods
Lactobacillus acidophilus	*	*
Lactobacillus brevis	*	*
Lactobacillus buchneri	*	*
Lactobacillus delbrueckii	*	*
Lactobacillus fermentum	*	*
Lactobacillus gasseri	*	-
Lactobacillus johnsonii	*	-
Lactobacillus paracasei	*	*
Lactobacillus plantarum	*	*
Lactobacillus reuteri	-	*
Lactobacillus rhamnosus	*	*
Lactobacillus ruminis	-	-
Lactobacillus salivarius	-	-
Bifidobacterium adolescentis	*	-
Bifidobacterium angulatum	-	-
Bifidobacterium bifidum	-	-
Bifidobacterium breve	-	-
Bifidobacterium catenulatum	-	-
Bifidobacterium dentium	*	-
Bifidobacterium infantis	-	-

(Table 3) cont.....

Microbial Species	Isolated From	
Bifidobacterium longum	-	-
Bifidobacterium pseudocatenulatum	-	-
Enterococcus faecalis	*	*
Enterococcus faecium	*	*

* Indicates the human gut microbial species which also isolated from clinical infections and/or fermented foods.

Over-Stimulation of the Immune System

Experiments in mice have shown that intestinal microbiota is essential for stimulating the immune system. The presence of intestinal microbiota is essential for various immune functions, such as antibody production, the establishment of oral tolerance to food antigens, and the formation of germinal centers within the oral follicles. The antagonistic effects of manipulation in the intestinal microbiota are particularly prominent in neonates where prolonged microbiota alteration can alter the immune response. The second group at risk of over-stimulation of the immune system due to probiotic consumption is pregnant women. During pregnancy, T cells' responses are drive to Th2 (since Th1 cytokines cause abortion), which is essential for maintaining fetal viability [88]. In *in-vitro* conditions, the probiotic strain of *Lactobacillus* suppressed Th2 cytokine responses and in some clinical studies increased the production of Th1 and interferon-gamma (IFNγ) cytokine, these effects can cause abortion [109]. However, there is currently no evidence of this effect and such a risk remains theoretical.

Transmission of Antibiotic-Resistance Genes

The bacterial antibiotic resistance properties can be inherent or acquired. The inherent resistance is a natural property and can regard as a species property. This type of resistance is non-transferable in most cases and is present in almost all members of a taxonomic group. On the contrary, there is the acquired resistance. The acquired resistance is due to the following: 1) accumulation of a mutation in DNA that leads to antibiotic resistance, 2) the acquired resistance genes from antibiotic-resistant bacteria. Resistance to antibiotics due to external DNA acquisition can transmit to other bacterial species or genera *via* plasmid or transposon [116]. In general, *Lactobacillus* species naturally show meaningful resistance to a wide range of antibiotics [117]. In most conditions, antibiotic resistance is not transferable. The *Lactobacillus* strains with non-transmissible antibiotic-resistance properties are usually considered safe microorganisms. Several *Lactobacilli* strains, such as *Lactobacillus rhamnosus* and *Lactobacillus casei* , are inherently resistant to vancomycin [117, 118]. Many *lactobacilli* strains are indigenously resistant to vancomycin, have been considered safe for use as probiotics [119]. Plasmid-mediated antibiotic resistance rarely occurs among *lactobacilli* [120], because antibiotic resistance genes can be phylogenetically transmitted between bacteria away from each other [121]. Most *bifidobacteria* are inherently resistant to nalidixic acid, neomycin, polymyxin B, kanamycin, gentamicin, streptomycin, and metronidazole [120]. In primary studies, vancomycin had an inhibitory effect against *bifidobacteria* [122]. However, recent studies have shown that vancomycin resistance is a general feature of all *bifidobacteria* [120].

Production of Toxic Metabolites

Production of Biogenic Amines

Biogenic amines are low molecular weight organic bases with a heterocyclic, aromatic, or aliphatic structure, and they can generate by decarboxylation of amino acids or amination and transamination of aldehydes and ketones. Since many lactic acid bacteria produce biogenic amines, starter cultures of lactic acid bacteria should lack decarboxylase enzymes to prevent the production of large amounts of biogenic amines in fermented foods [97, 123]. Other biogenic amines, such as putrescine, also have toxic effects [124]. Tryptamine and phenylethylamine are also considered to be undesirable amines due to their adverse effects [125]. Besides, secondary amines can react with nitrite in foods to produce carcinogenic nitrosamines [123]. Processed meat products are one of the food sources that can contain biogenic amines due to the use of poor quality raw materials, microbial contamination, and inappropriate conditions during the manufacturing process.

Production of D-Lactic Acid

Depending on the host and strains of consumed probiotics, harmful metabolic activities such as the induction of acidosis can occur through the production of D-lactic acid or the breakdown of bile salts. Such processes are due to the activity of the internal or external microbiota in the stomach and/or in the colon [98]. Human metabolism generally produces L-lactic acid isomer. A common feature in patients with D-lactate acidosis is excessive exposure to carbohydrates by D-lactate-producing bacteria. In these patients, recolonization with non-D-lactate producing bacteria is necessary. Overall, consumption of D-lactate-producing bacteria should be handled with greater caution, especially for patients at risk for metabolic acidosis, such as those undergoing intestinal surgery and those with irritable bowel syndrome as well as infants [126].

Limitations of Probiotic use in the Industry

In order to utilize probiotics in food and/or pharmaceutical products, these strains should keep their growth and proliferation abilities during the production process until consumption, and adding probiotic bacteria should not cause a loss of product quality [127]. Here we point out two major limitations of probiotic use in the industry.

Lack of Viability and Stability

The main challenge associated with the application of probiotic cultures in the creation of functional foods is to maintain their viability during the process. Probiotic microorganisms must be technologically suitable for use in food products. So that these microorganisms can maintain their viability and stability in the food products (on an industrial scale) and during preparation and consumption [128]. It is noteworthy that the growth and development of many probiotic bacteria are significantly affected during storage conditions when exposed to low pH, and also acidic conditions in the stomach [129]. It was also found that the viability and stability of probiotic bacteria are specific to each strain, and microencapsulation methods such as solvent evaporation have been successfully used to protect bacterial cells against damage caused by environmental conditions [130]. Other methods such as freeze-drying are also applied to confer long-term viability and stability [101, 131].

Alteration of the Flavor and Aroma of Probiotic Products

Probiotic cultures usually do not significantly alter the flavor and aroma of the products. The main concern is commonly associated with the cheeses containing *bifidobacteria* species due to these bacteria producing large amounts of acetic acid and lactic acid through the fructose-6-phosphate shunt pathway. The acetic acid in small amounts has a positive effect on the flavor of probiotic cheeses [127], but its high concentration is undesirable and loses the cheese's flavor.

Consequently, according to the stated cases, the use of probiotics is entirely safe only in healthy people, and also it should use with caution in children, elderly, pregnant women, and immunocompromised patients. Immature childhood infections appear to be high in these reports because they have poor immune systems. Immunocompromised individuals are more exposed to *lactobacillus* infections. Nevertheless, there are no infection reports with large statistical samples associated with *Bifidobacterium* spp. as well as animal investigations that demonstrated a low pathogenicity rate [132]. Several studies of probiotic-mediated infection suggested that individuals with pre-existing intestinal diseases are susceptible to infection. This evidence can consider as a general indicator of the use of probiotics. In recent years, scientists take a new approach to use probiotics in a non-viable form (currently known as postbiotics) to overcome the technological, economic, and clinical problems regarding the application of live probiotics.

CHAPTER 3

Postbiotics: A Solution to Leave Problems of the Production and Consumption of Probiotics

Abstract: The process of producing and distributing probiotics in the matrices of a wide variety of foods in the form of living cells has often been associate with difficulties. Several investigations have been doing to develop or optimize various approaches to maintain the viability of probiotic microbes. On the other hand, in recent years (mainly since 2010), a great deal of attention has been paid to using non-viable forms (postbiotics) bacteria as substitutes for probiotics. The term "postbiotic" refers to modified inactivated microbial cells, cell fractions, or cell metabolites that are naturally or synthetically generated by live probiotic cells and exert biological health-promoting effects to the host when administered in sufficient amounts. This chapter provides an overview of key concepts and main constituents of postbiotics, with emphasis on their biological activities.

Keywords: Ethyl phenyl sulfate, Flavonoids, Gut commensal bacteria, Indole, Long-chain fatty acids, Probiotic, Postbiotic, Prebiotics, Polyamines, Retinoic acid, Short-chain fatty acids, Trimethylamine-n-oxide.

The process of producing and distributing probiotics in the matrix of a wide range of fermented foods in the form of living cells has often been associated with problems. The consumption of probiotic products did not exert health effects on the host. Several investigations have been ongoing to develop or optimize methods to maintain the viability of probiotic microbes. In recent years (mainly since 2010), much attention has been paid to using non-living bacteria as substitutes for probiotics. Since the non-living forms of microbes do not fit into the definition of probiotics, scientists have used other terms such as "biogenic, abiotic, cell-free supernatant, paraprobiotic, metabiotic, ghost probiotic, pseudoprobiotic, and postbiotic" to define these non-viable and their biological metabolites [133]. Among them, the term "postbiotic" has received more attention in the scientific community [86, 87]. Postbiotics comprise inactivated microbial cells (non-living/dead cells), cell fractions (peptidoglycan-derived muropeptides, endo- and exo-polysaccharides, cell surface proteins , and teichoic acids), or cell

Amin Abbasi, Elham Sheykhsaran & Hossein Samadi Kafil

metabolites (short-chain fatty acids, organic acids, enzymes, and bacteriocins), and these bioactive components can improve overall host health (Fig. **3**) [18].

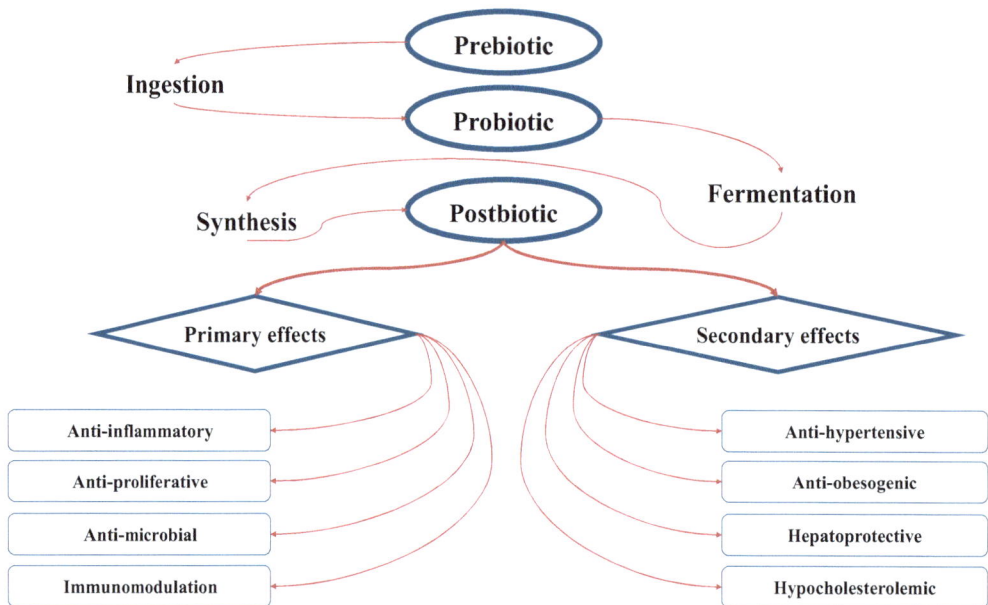

Fig. (3). Primary and secondary health effects of postbiotics. Prebiotics are non-digestible food ingredients in the small intestine but can easily consume *via* probiotics in the large colon. Small molecular weight metabolites/cell-wall constituents (<50, 50-100, and 100< kDa) (postbiotics) can be synthesized in the host intestinal environment by probiotic fermentation. These metabolites in the first step communicate with the gut environment and intestinal cells and exert their primary health effects (*e.g* ., anti-inflammatory, anti-proliferative, antimicrobial, immunomodulation) by modifying cellular processes, and subsequently in the second step with frequent consumption of probiotic/postbiotic products, confer further health effects (*e.g* ., anti-hypertensive, anti-obesogenic, hypocholesterolemic, hepatoprotective) *via* modifying metabolic pathways in the host.

Known and novel potential strains of probiotics may become a significant source of several low molecular weight bioactive molecules (LMWBM) (*e.g* ., short-chain and other fatty acids, polysaccharides, antimicrobial peptides, peptidoglycans, bacteriocins, biosurfactants, lipo and glycoproteins, teichoic acids, vitamins, antioxidants, peptides with different functional activity, nucleic acids, proteins comprising various enzymes and lectins, growth and coagulation elements, amino acids, inducers of defensin-like molecules, plasmalogens, phenol-containing compounds, co-factors, various signaling, and transport molecules, *etc.*) [133 - 136]. Numerous strains of symbiotic microorganisms can create sets of LMWBM. Hence they are considered as candidates for the creation of a general- /specific- target. High functionality and safety properties of the aforementioned biomolecules developed on their origin will fundamentally depend on the physicochemical features of microbial bioactive metabolites, their associations with other ingredients at the area of application, which can both amplify and hinder their bioactivity, rivalry in the scramble for particular transport proteins and /or absorption locality. The physiological and health status of the customer, daily diet, prescribed medication can substantially change the functionality and safety of microbial-derived bioactive constituents (postbiotics). Some groups of the LMWBMs derived from probiotic microorganisms (*e.g* ., organic acids, numerous peptides, microbial polysaccharides, amino acids, peptidoglycans, nucleic acids, nucleotides, antioxidants, vitamins, various co-factors, several types of transport and signaling biomolecules such as gas and other neurotransmitters) are presently being applied in industrial production of postbiotics [136]. For some symbiotic bacteria-derived components, goals, and outcomes have been set in both prokaryotic and eukaryotic cells. LMWBMs derived from endogenous and exogenous species can either transmit easily across the membranes of several microbial and eukaryotic cells (due to their lipophilic properties). Otherwise, they require particular cell -receptors and transporters for infiltration. They can work as precursors, co-substrates, mediators in various biochemical reactions and signaling pathways. Some of them have either signaling or only metabolic function. Pertaining on their active site, these biomolecules can be classified into molecular-level properties (*e.g* ., gene expression and replication, translation and transcription of genetic material), cell-level properties (cell surface, membranes, synthesis of energy and protein in mitochondria and ribosomes), inside the cell cytoplasm (in the position of organelles, nucleus, and cell ingredients), in extracellular space (at the position of vessels, synapses of neurons, the occurrence of metabolic reactions, exchange of extracellular information, *etc.*), in some tissues, organs, various physiological systems and the organism in general [86, 135]. The objectives for microbial biomolecules in mammalian organisms may characterize through the metagenome and meta-epigenome of microbial and eukaryotic cells, epigenetic regulation of specific gene expression and post-translational alteration of gene products, exchange of intracellular information such as quorum-sensing regulation, metabolic and behavioral reactions among gut microbial residents between the host and its symbiotic microbiota.

MAIN POSTBIOTIC CONSTITUENTS AND THEIR BIOLOGICAL ACTIVITIES

Large-scale genome-wide association investigations (GWAI) have shown various genetic influences on novel human diseases such as inflammatory, metabolic, and neurodegenerative diseases. Nevertheless, the instances in which GWAI have approached attaining impregnation with regard to the number of genetic relations to a specific sickness propose that human genetic factors are not solely responsible for the manifestation of these diseases. Moderately, lifestyle and environmental parameters possess a vital role in disease development. A key parameter of our conservational contact is demonstrated *via* daily nourishment and by gut commensal symbiotic microorganisms that exist in the digestive tract. It is noteworthy that the gut microbiota has been identifying to exert a significant role in human disease, and the precise mechanisms involved in host health benefits applied by these microorganisms have been widely studying during the past decade. Gut commensal bacteria can straightly involved in the host biological reactions *via* physical cell surface interactions or/and producing biomolecules, which enter the systemic blood circulation and exert influence on host physiology and health status. Current methodological advancements in the field of untargeted metabolomics have been applying in clearly defined clinical cohorts, which are associated with the mechanistic investigation in animal biological models that have described host disease-related gut microbial dysbiosis and their metabolome dysbiosis. Due to multiple functions of gut microbial-derived metabolites on vital physiologic metabolisms, the translational potential of these biomolecules for "postbiotic" therapies is tremendous [137, 138] (Fig. 4). These beneficial compounds can uniquely generate from the gut microbial fermentation process on a diet with indigestible nutrients (prebiotics) that moderate *via* intestinal microbes.

Trimethylamine-N-Oxide (TMAO)

TMAO is considering an example of metabolites derived from gut microbial metabolism that has a significant potential application. TMAO is associated with an extensive variety of chronic disorders. In addition to metabolic and cardiovascular diseases, such as myocardial infarction, stroke, atherosclerosis, and type 2 diabetes [139 - 143], some investigations defined TMAO as a possible prognostic biomarker of end-stage renal and chronic kidney disease [144], while inconsistent results were newly published [145]. It has been demonstrating that in patients with Alzheimer's disease and minor cognitive disorder, TMAO is incremented in the cerebrospinal fluid [146]. TMAO is commonly generating through a diet-originated meta-organismal path. Egg, red meat, milk, and some seafood are full of the lipid phosphatidylcholine, which considers a substantial foundation of the vital nutrient choline in omnivores. Choline and other TMA-comprising species (betaine, L-carnitine) are catabolized through gut microbial TMA lyases and produce the gas form of TMA [147]. The absorbed TMA by the intestinal cells enters the blood circulation, then metabolized to TMAO *via* the hepatic flavin monooxygenase3 (FMO3) [148]. Generation of TMAO from dietary choline occurs by means of a healthy gut microbiome. In this regard, the TMAO generation, in germ-free mice, after administration of deuterium-labeled PC was unsuccessful. However, the d9 isotopomer of TMAO was positively generating in the control group [149]. TMAO stimulates changes in sterol and cholesterol (diminutions in reverse cholesterol transport) metabolism besides, it can alter bile acid composition [150, 151]. Though the receptor sites for TMAO are not yet recognized, this metabolite was shown to promote thrombosis risk and platelet hyperreactivity [152].

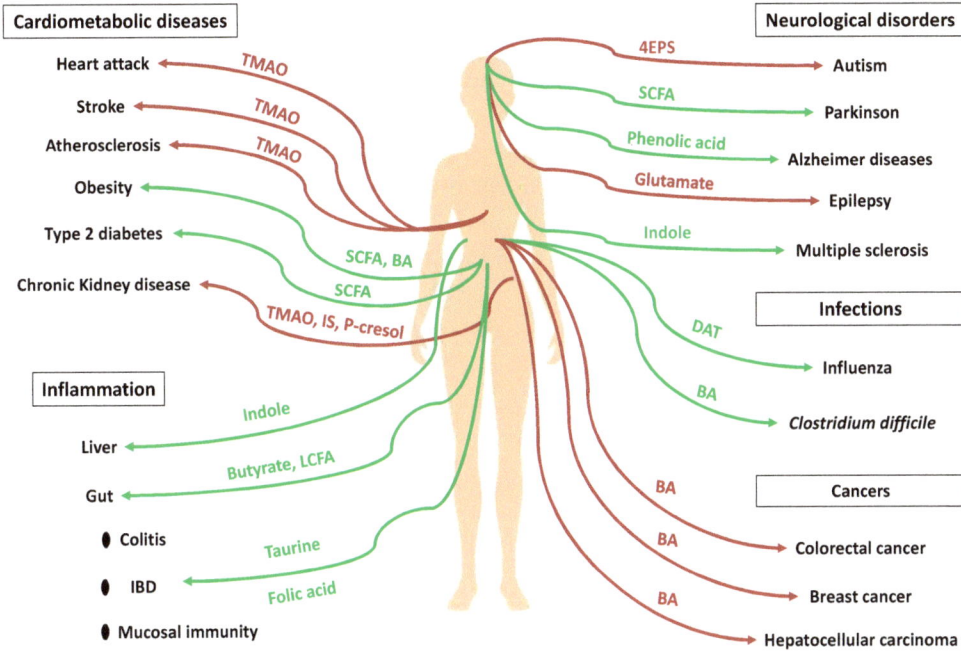

Fig. (4). The effect of bioactive compounds produced by gut microbiome in some disorders. Arrows signify a positive (green) or negative (red) role for particular gut microbiome- related metabolites in various diseases. TMAO: Trimethylamine-N-oxide. SCFA: short- chain fatty acids. BA: Bile acid. IS: Indoxyl sulfate. LCFA: Long-chain fatty acids. 4EPS: 4-ethylphenylsulfate. DAT: desaminotyrosine. IBD: inflammatory bowel disease.

Wang *et al.*, (2015), studied the influence of targeted inhibition of the first step in TMAO production, gut commensal microbial TMA generation, on diet-stimulated atherosclerosis. They concluded that targeting the gut microbial generation of TMA particularly and non-lethal microbial inhibitors overall may confer as a possible therapeutic strategy for the treatment of cardiometabolic diseases [153]. This work characterizes a proof of concept that a gut microbiome-related enzymatic system can be aimed to generate novel therapeutic compounds for human diseases. Due to this, TMAO can be recognized as a reason rather than a result of the disease- stimulating property [154], the subsequent phase to targeted clinical application will be to found the safety profile, effectiveness, and biochemical and physiologic effects (pharmacodynamics) for this inhibitor in the host.

Short-Chain Fatty Acids (SCFAs)

SCFAs are considering the main bioactive compounds produced in the intestine. Butyrate, propionate, and acetate are generating by gut bacterial fermentation of non-digestible dietary fibers (prebiotics) [155]. These biomolecules are recognizing by various G-protein coupled receptors (GPRs) (also characterized as free fatty acid receptors (FFARs) and the intracellular receptor PPARγ) of the intestinal cells. Additionally, SCFAs can similarly adjust various cellular responses by the prohibition of histone deacetylases (HDACs). SCFAs exert beneficial effects on the host through the down-regulation of pro-inflammatory mediators and regulatory macrophage and T (Treg) cell differentiation. These properties significantly assistance in maintaining a balance between intestinal inflammation and immunity [155 - 158]. Besides, SCFAs have been demonstrating to modify T cell homeostasis, promote IgA responses, moderate insulin sensitivity, fat accumulation, promote neurogenesis, and modified hematopoiesis [159 - 164]. There has been growing interest to discover their potentially therapeutic functions in various acute and chronic diseases due to their principal role in establishing gut eubiosis, shaping the metabolism and immune system. SCFAs are being applied in randomized controlled trials (RCTs) to remedy a variety of disorders influencing gastrointestinal health, neurological performances, and metabolism. Modifications in the gut microbiome in terms of composition and balance can be associated with the appearance of fatness, inflammatory disorders such as inflammatory bowel disease (IBD), and diabetes [165]. Lipid metabolism and blood glucose control are remarkably engaged in metabolic disorders, and some of the SCFAs, such as butyrate, have been revealed to positively affected these activities [166]. A clinical study indicated that enema administration of SCFA (butyrate) in individuals in remission from irritable bowel syndrome (IBS) or ulcerative colitis exert slight effects [167]. The potential therapeutic function of SCFAs is also being surveying for the gut-brain axis. Butyrate as a cellular energy source, G-protein coupled receptors activator, and HDAC inhibitor has been suggesting moderate common symptoms in autism, Alzheimer's, Huntington's, schizophrenia, and Parkinson's [168 - 173]. Some clinical trials are ongoing to evaluate butyrate's biological properties of cognitive performance in individuals with schizophrenia, especially regarding its epigenetic regulation of inflammation (NCT03010865). Presently, a mixture of various SCFAs is being investigated for their key role in affective some nervous system processing such as fear, emotions, and stress (NCT03688854). Nevertheless, these discussed clinical studies exploited SCFAs straightly as therapeutic agents, recently, there is growing attention in the utilization of prebiotics as a raw material, which can be applied by the gut microbiota to produce SCFAs [171 - 174].

Long-Chain Fatty Acids (LCFAs)

LCFAs have long been applying as nutritional supplementation, either as perilla oil or linseed comprising linoleic acid and fish oils comprising omega-6 and omega-3 fatty acids (FA). LCFAs are crucial nutrients for the host, as mammals cannot produce them, these essential nutrients are mainly gained through diet and ultimately metabolized to produce bioactive lipid mediators. These have been reported to moderate inflammation by the diminution of inflammatory cytokines or the diminution of blood pressure (arachidonic acid) [175, 176]. Currently, LCFAs have been identifying as gut microbial metabolites. Several conjugated linoleic acids (CLAs), hydroxy FA, and oxy FA are producing *via* intestinal commensal bacteria: *Enterococcus faecalis, Bacteroides thetaiotaomicron,* and *Lactobacillus plantarum* [177]. On the other hand, it has been revealed that linoleic acids formed by gut microbes can stimulate intracellular PPARγ receptors in macrophages [178]. However, similarly strengthening intestinal epithelial barrier integrity by up-regulation of tight junctions. In particular, 10-hydroxy-c-s-12 octadecenoic acid (HYA) is one CLA which due to its biological activity has been described as a promising therapeutic tool for the reinforcement of epithelial barrier totality [179, 180]. Omega acids have long been revealed that it is beneficial to the brain and heart function, and currently, with collecting evidence of gut microbial-derived LCFAs, recent investigations discover using CLAs in therapy as postbiotics. Furthermore, some results of RCTs have shown the capability of CLA to restrict body fat mass in healthy, and overweight subjects probably by regulation of fatty acid biotransformation [181, 182]. Another investigation suggested that CLAs applied as an oral complement with fiber and vitamin could be efficacious as adjuvant therapy in ulcerative colitis [183].

4-Ethyl Phenyl Sulfate (4-EPS)

4-Ethyl Phenyl Sulfate (4-EPS) 4-EPS is a bio-product derived from the final stage of fermentation, assumed to be a uremic toxin. Germ-free and pathogen-free mice obviously possess a very low amount of 4-EPS. Scientists' attention to this metabolite arises from a report that demonstrated a significant rise in 4-EPS in the model of maternal immune activation (MIA) in rats with autism spectrum disorder (ASD). These high levels of 4-EPS are associated with behavioral irregularities. Administration of *B. fragilis* improved unfavorable effect signifying the possible application of probiotic and postbiotic therapies for ASD [184].

Indole

Amino-acid metabolism from the gut commensal microbiome characterizes as the base source of biomolecules to the host [185]. Tryptophanase plays an important role in the catalysis of the essential amino acid tryptophan to indole, which is uniquely encoding in microbial genomes [186]. Some tryptophan byproducts such as indole-3-aldehyde converted by *Lactobacillus*-encoded tryptophanase or 3-indole propionic acid (IPA) from *Clostridium sporogenes* are identifying by the aryl hydrocarbon receptor. Aryl hydrocarbon receptor is a ligand-dependent transcription factor that incorporates ecological, nutritional, microbial, and metabolic indications to regulate intricate transcriptional programs in a ligand-, cell type-, and context-specific method [187]. Gut epithelial cell-specific elimination of aryl hydrocarbon receptor results in fracture to control *C. rodentium* infection [188]. Aryl hydrocarbon receptor also facilitates the influence of the gut microbiome on intra-epithelial lymphocytes [189]. In this regard, Zelante *et al.*, (2013), described a metabolic pathway that accord to it, tryptophan metabolites from the microbiota balance mucosal reactivity in mice model. Indole-3-aldehyde signaling by aryl hydrocarbon receptor facilitates IL- 22 generation in type 3 innate lymphoid cells under infection condition stimulated *via Candida albicans*. The authors concluded that the microbiota-aryl hydrocarbon receptor axis might characterize an important approach followed by coevolutive commensalism for well-tuning host mucosal reactivity contingent on tryptophan catabolism [190]. Further gut commensal microbiome-derived bioactive compounds are also endowed with aryl hydrocarbon receptor agonistic properties, such as indole-3- aldehyde, indole-3- acetyl aldehyde, 2-(1′H-indoe-3′-carbonyl)-thiazole-4-carboxylic acid methyl ester (ITE), 3-methylindole, and indole-3-acetic acid. Indole metabolites can also thwart harmful inflammation in LPS-induced hepatitis (liver inflammation) by the regulation of the NLRP3 pathway [191].

In a preclinical model of multiple sclerosis (experimental autoimmune encephalomyelitis), microbial-derived indole metabolites regulated central nervous system inflammation by the diminution of the pathogenic function of astrocytes [192 - 194]. In neurodegenerative diseases, the cerebellar syndrome has been associating with a neurochemical shortage of 5- hydroxytryptamine. Present clinical trials will assess indole-3-propionic acid supplementation, a 5-hydroxytryptamine precursor, as a promising therapeutic approach for multiple sclerosis and Friedreich's ataxia. Indole can transform into indoxyl and indoxyl sulfate through host hepatic oxidases (CYP2E1 and SULT1A1) . Indoxyl sulfate is supposed to be a "uremic toxin", whose elimination from the body through renal excretion is reduced in kidney disease [195]. Indoxyl sulfate is likely considering a possible vascular toxin that can increase the proliferation of vascular smooth muscle cells, stimulate oxidative stress in endothelial cells, and impressively participate in the pathophysiology of sarcopenia and atherosclerosis in individuals with the renal disorder [195, 196].

Numerous efforts to moderate indole metabolites for therapeutic targets are under study. *Arabinoxylan oligosaccharides* are considering the non-digestible carbohydrates (prebiotic) with significant health-stimulating features that promote the growth and development of specific intestinal bacteria, especially *Bifidobacteria*. *Arabinoxylan oligosaccharides* are investigating in chronic kidney disorder for lowering indole byproducts (indoxyl sulfate). An alternative to *Arabinoxylan oligosaccharides* is AST-120 (kremezin; Kureha Chemical, Tokyo, Japan) is an oral globular carbonaceous adsorbent, which has been approved for clinical application in Japanese chronic kidney disease patients in 1991. AST-120 adsorbs indole and inhibits indoxyl sulfate generation as well as it's presently studied in clinical trials as a potential therapeutic tool for chronic kidney disease. A substitute therapeutic approach would be to straightly hinder aryl hydrocarbon receptor through delivering antagonists single and/or in nanoparticles as well as design enzyme enhanced to metabolize aryl hydrocarbon receptor agonists [187].

Para-cresol (P-cresol or 4-methyl phenol) an isomer of o-cresol and m-cresol, and its derivative p-cresyl sulfate, is another gut microbial metabolite from protein fermentation that naturally not formed by host enzymes [197]. It is assumed to promote vascular calcification [198], to modify endothelial function [199], the pathogenesis of *Clostridium difficile* infection, and ulcerative colitis [200], and has been related to augmented mortality in hemodialysis patients [201]. Although increased daily high-fat diet consumption in healthy individuals increases indole and p-cresol [202], a daily dietary approach with oligofructose-enriched inulin significantly participates in a minor production of protein fermentation metabolites and establishes a noteworthy enhancement for chronic kidney disease patients [203, 204]. *Arabinoxylan oligosaccharides* consumption meaningfully increases the number of fecal *bifidobacteria* and diminishes urinary p-cresol excretion [205].

Other Protein-Derived Metabolites

Taurine is an amino sulfonic acid that occurs naturally in the body and is predominantly concentrates in the eyes, brain, heart, and muscle tissues. Unlike most other amino acids, it is not applying to form proteins. Taurine levels are regulated through de-conjugation of primary bile acids by gut commensal bacteria [206, 207], triggering an increment in luminal taurine levels. Taurine was detected to stimulate NLRP6 inflammasome signaling and subsequently suggested to regulate IBD [208]. Taurine is similarly being investigating as a defensive substance in diabetes and bowel cancer. One investigation evaluates the quantity of sulfidogenic microbes in African Americans with daily nourishments low or rich in taurine to perceive risk features for bowel cancer, such as inflammation markers, oxidative stress, and primary and secondary bile acid pools [209]. In the meantime, two clinical trials applied taurine to treat vascular side-effects in diabetes that may arise by oxidative stress (NCT03410537, NCT01226537).

The defensive properties of the ketogenic diet (a high-fat, adequate-protein, low-carbohydrate diet) have been revealed to be mediated *via* the gut commensal microbiome through the decrement of amino acid y-glutamylation, eventually leading to augmented GABA/glutamate content in the brain [210].

Desaminotyrosine (4-hydroxy phenyl propionic acid) is a by-product of tyrosine metabolism and obviously existent in mammalian urine. The results from a recent investigation indicated that an intact intestinal microbiota as well as especially the existence of *Clostridium orbiscendens* is essential for detectable desaminotyrosine levels in the serum and feces [211]. Decrement of desaminotyrosine generation was related to augmenting vulnerability to viral infection, due to suboptimal reinforcement of the type I interferon signaling loop. Yet, no registered clinical trials are evaluating the translation of these outcomes to the clinic.

Imidazole propionate is newly recognizing as a microbial-produced histidine-derived metabolite that exerts a vital role in the pathophysiology of type 2 diabetes. Higher levels of Imidazole propionate tend to be found in type 2 diabetes patients compared to healthy individuals and in turn lead to the deterioration of the insulin signaling at the level of insulin receptor substrate through activating p38y MAPK, which stimulates p62 phosphorylation as well as activates the mechanistic target of rapamycin complex 1 (mTORC1) [212]. Consequently, clinical trials will assess various diets (low-protein against high-protein) that can hinder imidazole propionate generation (NCT03732690).

Polyamines

Polyamines have been associating with the modulation of inflammation pathways and the stimulation of inflammatory bowel diseases (*e.g* . colitis) [208]. Some metabolites such as spermidine (is a polyamine compound found in ribosomes and living tissues), are either produced *via* the gut microbiota, *via* the host, or consumed by the daily diet, and have multiple properties on numerous diverse tissues [213]. Spermine is a biogenic polyamine generated from spermidine. It is found in an extensive range of organisms and tissues and is a vital growth factor in some bacteria. Spermine can significantly influence the NLRP6 inflammasome pathway, which in turn changes gut microbial composition. Indeed, some members of the *Lactobacillus* genus possess polyamine production by biosynthetic and transport pathways of spermine [208]. Spermine- generated by decarboxylation of amino acids (*e.g* . ornithine) inhibits NLRP6 inflammasome assembly and diminishes colonic IL-18 levels. In individuals with inflammatory bowel disease and mice model with chronic DSS-stimulated colitis, augmented levels of the polyamine precursor spermidine were detected [214]. Insights into a potential role for polyamine suppression as a practical approach against IBD in patients require clinical trials with a large statistical society [215].

Gut microbiome-related polyamines have also been associating with the adjustment of epithelial circadian rhythms [216]. Daily fluctuations affect the gut microbiome and intestinal polyamine levels [216, 217]. Modification of polyamine rhythms is related to clock dysfunction [218], and therefore regulation of intestinal polyamine levels might provide a reasonable strategy to adjusting transcriptional fluctuations in intestinal epithelial cells.

Retinoic Acid

Retinoic acid (is a member of the over 4000-strong family of retinoids, which are compounds derived from retinol or dietary vitamin A), has been involved fundamentally in the regulation and development of the immune system. Retinoic acid quantity in the intestinal is in turn sustained through *Clostridia* commensal bacteria *via* inhibition of retinol dehydrogenase 7 in epithelial cells [219]. Retinoic acid has been revealed to participate in the moderation of immune system responses by the production of IgA [161]. Furthermore, retinoic acid sustains T-cell immunity by regulatory T cell differentiation and T helper 17 cell regulation [220]. The result of studies demonstrated that the shortages in retinoic acid quantity or its receptors have been linked with some chronic disease states such as IBD, and colitis-associated colon cancer [221]. Due to numerous scientific reports involving retinoic acid's role in T cell development, all-trans-retinoic acid is discovering as a promising treatment in diseases of uncontrolled immune situations such as rheumatoid arthritis, cancer, auto-immune disorders, and thrombocytopenia [222 - 225]. Up to now, there has been one finished Phase 2 study establishing that individuals with primary immune thrombocytopenia treated with all-trans-retinoic acid indicated promoted response of sustained platelet levels (NCT01667263). All trans-retinoic acid is also presently applied to treat leukemia and acne under the name tretinoin. However, its precise mechanism is still presently unidentified. Additional investigations are necessary to explore the application of retinoic acid in all-trans-retinoic acid form or 13-cis retinoic form in the regulation of inflammation in the intestinal.

Bile Acids

Primary bile acids, cholic acid, and chenodeoxycholic acid are produced in the liver tissue from cholesterol *via* hepatocytes and characterize more than 75% of the body's total bile acids content. Gut commensal bacteria (in the small and large intestine), the bacterial dehydrogenation, 7α- dehydroxylation, epimerization, and deconjugation, of the primary bile acids, generates the "secondary" bile acids.

Cholic acid is transformed to dihydroxy deoxycholic acid and chenodeoxycholic acid to the mono hydroxy lithocholic acid. Gut bacteria can more metabolize 7a-oxo- lithocholic acid to "tertiary" bile acid, dihydroxy ursodeoxycholic acid [226]. Bile acids play the main role in sustaining cholesterol homeostasis by the emulsification and absorption of lipids. Gut bacteria with bile salt hydrolase properties, such as *Clostridium*, and *Lactobacillus* simplify several aspects of bile acid metabolism such as dehydrogenation, dihydroxylation, and deconjugation [227, 228]. Germ-free mice possess higher general bile acid levels, typically ursodeoxycholic acid, also bigger gallbladders due to stimulation of the transmembrane G protein-coupled receptor 5 pathway [229]. Cold temperature exposure prompts the conversion of cholesterol to bile acids in the liver tissue, modifies gut microbiome composition, induces lipoprotein processing in brown adipose tissue, and produces heat in mice model [230].

The results from recent investigations have specified that ursodeoxycholic acid develops insulin sensitivity and stimulates weight loss in individuals with type 2 diabetes (NCT02033876). It also possesses a vital role in combating infection. Ursodeoxycholic acid suppressed the growth and development of *Clostridium difficile* in fecal specimens from individuals with frequent *C. difficile* infections and was efficacious in treating a case with *C. difficile*-related pouchitis [231]. A clinical study will aim to accredit this outcome by the administration of urs ursodiol idol/ ursodeoxycholic acid to cases with frequent *C. difficile* infections (NCT02748616). Moreover, a higher quantity of deoxycholic acid is related to colonic crypt renewal after injuring [232]. Deoxycholic acid used farnesoid X receptor (FXR) to suppress prostaglandin E2 production (a constituent that hinders crypt repair), so developing wound repair [232].

Furthermore, some investigations have centralized on hindering secondary bile acids as a form of treatment. Numerous studies have shown high concentrations of secondary bile acids to augmented risk for different forms of cancer (liver, pancreatic, and colorectal cancer) and characterized their capability to stimulate cell death as well as DNA mutations. In this regard, using the murine model of liver cancer, Ma *et al.*, (2018), reported that the administration of secondary bile acids (*e.g* . ω-muricholic acid) diminished natural killer T cell agglomeration and diminished CXCL16 expression, thus reversing the antitumor properties of primary bile acids [233]. Further scientific works have reported meaningfully higher deoxycholic acid levels in colorectal cancer individuals and augmented hepatocellular carcinoma risk with elevated deoxycholic acid levels [234, 235]. Nevertheless, taking down deoxycholic acid levels (using either ursodeoxycholic acid or difructose anhydride III) diminished hepatocellular carcinoma progress in obese mice [235].

Flavonoids

Flavonoids are a class of polyphenolic plant and fungus secondary metabolites that are recognized to have a vast variety of biological properties such as protective functions on vascular endothelial cells, antioxidant effects, anti-proliferative as well as anti-carcinogenic effects. These compounds are a particular subclass within the major set of polyphenols, and the gut microbiota possesses a noteworthy function in flavonoid metabolism [236]. Gut commensal microbiota participates in both the fermentation and hydrolysis of consumed flavonoids [237], and antibiotics treated or germ-free mice, therefore, have high quantities of flavonoids in their intestines [238]. For instance, *Bacteroides uniform* and *Bacteroides distasonis* are two of numerous microbial species that are directly involved in the hydrolysis of polyphenol compounds. Consequently, the gut microbiota is vital to simplifying these digestive processes, but the flavonoids and polyphenols themselves may likewise modify gut microbiota composition and balances. For instance, a study discovered that the flavonoids quercetin and rutin can hinder the growth of *Serratia marcescens* and *E. coli* [239].

Besides, flavonoids seem to have disease-improving properties in obese mice. Liu *et al.*, (2017), studied molecular factors involved in the hypolipidemic and hypoglycemic properties of the flavonoid-rich extract from Paulownia fortunei flowers (EPF) in obese mice fed a high-fat diet (HFD). They reported a significant diminution in hepatic steatosis, hyperlipidemia, and insulin resistance in HFD mice after oral gavage with an EPF. In this study, the protective properties of EPF were possibly related to reducing SREBP-1c, HMGCR, and FAS expressions and the increase in phosphor-IRS-1 and CPT1 expression. The authors concluded that EPF might be a potential natural candidate for the prevention and/or treatment of overweight, hepatic, and metabolic-associated modifications prompted by HFD [240]. Clinical studies aimed at assessing the postbiotic properties of polyphenols produced from the dietary plant Virgin Olive Oil and Red Wine (NCT03101436) in diabetic and obese individuals. Furthermore, the flavonoid-metabolizing properties of the intestinal microbiota become physiologically pertinent in the post-obesity state [241]. In this regard, in a regaining of weight post-dieting mouse model, Thaiss *et al.*, (2016), established that incessant post-obesity microbiome modifications sustained a scarcity of the two flavonoids apigenin and naringenin in the intestine [238]. Postbiotic supplementation of these compounds augmented host energy expenditure and improved relapsing obesity.

Furthermore, some investigations have described that flavonoids like luteolin possess significant antioxidant properties that can hinder mast cells, which are known to participate in the inflammatory pathway. In another study, Weng *et al.*,

(2015), investigated the capability of luteolin and its novel structural analog 3',4',5,7-tetra methoxy luteolin (methlut) to hinder human mast cell moderator expression and release *in vitro* and *in vivo*. They established that methlut suppressed the release of inflammatory mediators including histamine secretion, tumor necrosis factor (TNF), and beta-hexosaminidase from mast cells, as well as concluded that methlut is a promising mast cell inhibitor for the treatment of inflammatory and allergic conditions [242]. On the other hand, flavonoids seem to have valuable therapeutical effects among several types of brain-related disorders and diseases. For instance, flavonoids have revealed favorable outcomes in Alzheimer's disease. Grape-derived polyphenolics, a strong antioxidant, have been described to hinder amyloid-β (Abeta) oligomerization and diminish cognitive deterioration in a mouse model of Alzheimer's disease [243]. Consequently, the results from discussed studies specify that moderating the gut microbiome to increase gut flavonoid quantities might be helpful for an extensive range of conditions.

N-Acyl Amides

N-acyl amides are bioactive lipids that play several roles in biological systems such as cell-to-cell communication. These N-acyl amino acids are categorizing *via* unsaturated fatty acyl chains, medium-chain, and neutral amino acid head groups. Commendamide (*N*-acyl-3- hydroxy palmitoyl -glycine) is a natural product from the gut microbiome that can commonly identify through functional metagenomic screening for nuclear factor NF-kB activators. It looks like long-chain N- acyl-amides and activates a G-protein coupled receptor G2A/GPR132 as mammalian signaling molecules involved in atherosclerosis and autoimmunity [244]. Genes anticipated to encode like lipids were more recognized, produced, and inserted into *E. coli*. These lipids were then established *versus* GPCR. The microbial lipid N-acyl serinol is analogous to a host ligand for GPR119, which once operated induces glucagon-like peptide-1 release from the gut L-cells, and controlled metabolic hormone function and glucose homeostasis. Parallel outcomes were found when N-acyl serinol is fed to mice [245]. No registered clinical study is available to assess its potential translation to human pathologies [246].

The instances discussed here demonstrate the functional flexibility of biomolecules that are generated or modulated by the gut microbiome. While the concept of modifying the concentrations of these biomolecules for therapeutic purposes is instinctive and corresponding with decades of practice in the field of pharmacology, we believe that several obstacles need to overcome on the path toward successful use of postbiotics as therapeutic modalities. In conclusion, based on the dynamic nature of the microbiome and its disease relevance, optimal concentrations of postbiotics might be highly context-dependent. Furthermore, there is a need for additional investigations to determine the optimal timing for interventions base on microbial metabolites in disease development. Despite impediments, targeting the meta-organismal pathways involved in the generation and signaling of microbiome-associated metabolites offers a vast and intact opportunity to control sickness sensibility.

CHAPTER 4

Main Methods for the Preparation of Postbiotics

Abstract: Fermentation process is the fundamental and natural way to produce postbiotics. In this process, different microbial strains exploit prebiotics to generate a wide variety of postbiotics with several health-promoting effects (*e.g.*, antimicrobial, antioxidant, anticancer, *etc* .), by natural methods or in response to environmental conditions. Further, postbiotics play a substantial role in the enrichment of the food matrix. In addition to the natural methods in postbiotics production, different laboratory methods can be used to produce a purer form and with high functionality in fermented and non-fermented food, which in turn improves their nutritional values, shelf-life, and health-beneficial effects in consumers. This chapter will discuss the main laboratory postbiotic production process, with emphasis on their quality controls.

Keywords: Fermentation process, Genome-scale metabolic model, Heat inactivation, High pressure, Ionizing radiation, Lactic acid bacteria, Postbiotics, Quality control, Sonication, Ultraviolet.

MAIN POSTBIOTIC PRODUCER MICROBIAL CELLS

Probiotic strains are frequently affiliated with lactic acid bacteria (LAB), some yeast strains [247], and/or Gram-negative bacteria (*e.g* ., *Escherichia coli* Nissle 1917) [248]. LAB has the capability to utilize complex carbohydrates (*e.g.*, lactose, sucrose, fructose, and other sugars) and convert them to lactic acid through the lactic acid fermentation process. They are obligate or facultative anaerobes, which can tolerate and grow in anaerobic conditions. Technologically significant genera consist of *Lactobacillus*, *Lactococcus*, *Bifidobacteria*, *Pediococcus*, *Streptococcus*, and *Leuconostoc*.

Lactobacillus is the key genera of LAB and can possess a vital role in modulating the gut microbiome balances. These bacteria can be either homo- and/or hetero-fermentative and extensively applied in the vegetable and dairy fermentation process. In the host gut microbiome, *lactobacilli* establish a small niche in the ecosystem. For instance, *L. casei*, *L. plantarum*, and *L. acidophilus* are allochthonous strains and insist on the gastrointestinal tract through ongoing administration [249]. *Lactobacilli* are resilient to the harsh conditions of digestive

Amin Abbasi, Elham Sheykhsaran & Hossein Samadi Kafil

systems such as gastric acids and bile salts. As probiotics when consumed, *lactobacilli* rival with other pathogenic germs for communicating to epithelial cells, nutrients, colonization [250], and to promote barrier function [251, 252]. Moghadam *et al.* [253] described that six strains of *L. plantarum* (TL1, UL4, RI11, RS5, RG11, and RG14), isolated and identified from Malaysian fermented foods [254], ensconce two types of bacteriocin structural genes, namely plantaricin EF and W. This specifies that these *lactobacilli* strain are the unique source to produce bacteriocin, presenting extensive inhibitory properties [255, 256]. According to a study conducted by Tai *et al.* [257], the concurrent attendance of two types of bacteriocin structural genes within a probiotic cell has not been described elsewhere. Notwithstanding these strains being much resembled at the genomic level, random amplified polymorphic DNA (RAPD) analysis and short non-transcribed spacer (NGS) region at 16Se23S region analysis indicated different strain contradistinction. *plw* and *plnEF* loci pertain to two various types of bacteriocin molecules. Plantaricin EF and plantaricin W pertain to type II and class I bacteriocins, respectively. Remarkably, the UL4-*plnEF* locus is a composite from the J51-*plnEF* locus and *lactobacilli* strain JDM1-*plnEF* locus in terms of organization and genetic composition [257, 258].

Consequently, for postbiotics, at least a mixture of two treatments is required to interrupt the microbial membrane to attain the intracellular and/or cell-wall bioactive molecules in the form of fragments. However, in some cases, the resulting combination could contain non-viable cells and postbiotics concurrently; therefore, further stages such as microfiltration, are required to remove intact microbial cells and recover the postbiotic components. Meantime, for obtaining postbiotic components *via* parent cells, centrifugation and/or filtration processes are applied to eliminate the viable microbial cells from the culture medium [258].

THE MAIN LABORATORY POSTBIOTIC PRODUCTION PROCESS

The Primary Step (Inactivation Methods) in the Postbiotic Production Process

Postbiotics can be gained through inactivating viable probiotic cells by different laboratory methods. The most extensively applied manners are heat inactivation (HI), high pressure (HP) technique, ionizing radiation (IR), sonication (S), and inactivation by ultraviolet (UV) rays (Fig. **5**) [133]. The typical manners for inactivation of viable probiotic cells are HI, formalin inactivation (FI), UV treatment, and S. Among these manners, HI is the most commonly applied manner for postbiotic preparation. In the primary step, these methods lead to the death of probiotic cells, and each method has various modes of action for inactivation. Though, it is to be noted that the inactivation manner should have the capability to maintain in postbiotics the helpful characteristics of the probiotic cells (Table **4**) [259].

Table 4. The main methods of elimination of live starter microorganisms, the devastation of microbial suspensions, and isolation of postbiotic metabolites.

Item No.	Methods
1	Frequent freezing and thawing
2	Applying enzymes with specific activity against microbial cell walls, membranes, intracellular structures
3	Mechanical destruction
4	Ionizing radiation
5	Ultrasound damaging
6	Microwave radiation
7	Ultraviolet radiation
8	Utilizing liquid carbon dioxide for inactivation of microorganism suspensions and extraction of cell components and metabolite compounds
9	Various methods of ultrafiltration of whole and destroyed cell suspensions
10	Different kinds of dialysis, the use of ion-exchange resins
11	Cell destructive by chemical mediators (for example, exposure to acids)
12	High hydrostatic pressure
13	Supercritical water extraction

Heat Inactivation (HI)

The frequently applied procedure to inactivate microbial cells is the use of heat for a specified period. The high temperature in HI manner can significantly influence various components of the cell structure of microbial cells of which loss of nutrients and ions, disruption of membrane integrity, inactivation of essential enzymes and coagulation of protein, rupture of DNA filaments, ribosome aggregation are of specific relevance [260]. Nevertheless, the performance of HI manner may be impressed *via* several parameters such as the strains of parent probiotic cells, the type of growth medium and its pH, water activity, stage of growth, vegetative or spore form of microorganisms, and mode of heating, among others [261]. HI-treated microbial cultures are a source of various soluble biomolecules such as fragments of cell-wall ingredients and microbial DNA [262]. It has been described that the CpG motif of microbial DNA remains conserved even in non-viable bacteria after HI-treatment [263]. Stimulation of immune function *via* bacterial CpG motif and several cell-wall constituents has mostly been described [263].

Therefore, HI-treated bacteria can induce specific immune responses through such mechanisms. From another point of view, cell roughness, adhesion, and coarseness characteristics are vital features of probiotic cells that can undesirably influence immunity and other helpful properties [264, 265]. HI, manner can influence the functional characteristics of microbial cells (increase the cell roughness and coarseness, as well as decrease the adhesion ability), which in turn, can undesirably impact the beneficial properties of postbiotics. Furthermore, modification of such attributes of postbiotics is strain-dependent [266]. These indicate that a well understanding of the science on inactivation state and the anticipated helpful properties is vital for postbiotics production [133]. For instance, as far as research in aquaculture area is interested, production of postbiotics has been done *via* using various HI conditions including 60°C for 30 min [267], 60°C for 1 h [268, 269], 65°C for 30 min [270], 75°C for 60 min [271], 80°C for 30 min [272], 80°C for 60 min [273], 95°C for 60 min [274], keeping probiotic bacteria in boiling water for 1–2 h [275, 276], and 150 °C for 15 min [277].

UV Inactivation (UV)

Ultraviolet rays are a form of electromagnetic non-ionizing radiation non-ionizing irradiance with a wavelength from 200 to 400 nm and confer significant microbicide activities. This spectrum divided into three areas (short-wave UV (200 to 280 nm), medium-wave UV (280 to 320 nm), and long-wave UV (320 to 400 nm)), in which the short-wave area possess higher microbicide properties and/or efficiently inactivate an extensive variety of microbial cells and spores [278, 279]. Contact ultraviolet rays lead to the denaturation of microbial protein and the generation of DNA photoproducts. The main mechanisms of UV manner can be associated with the generation of dimer between adjoining pyrimidine molecules on the same DNA strand that leads to discontinuity of transcription and translation processes, consequently, result in mutagenesis and cell death [280]. Only a few investigations have been performed on UV rays induced inactivation of probiotic cells where a UV exposition time of 2.5 h was applied for inactivation [268, 269, 281].

Formalin Inactivation (FI)

Formalin also is one of the recommended practices applied to deactivate probiotic microbial cells [282]. This manner has been utilized by numerous investigators using a 37% aqueous solution of formaldehyde gas with changeable time and temperature. In this manner, the main mechanism of action is founded on alkylating the hoop nitrogen atoms of purine bases, sulfhydryl, and amino sulfhydryl groups of proteins [283]. Probiotic cells were deactivated *via* the addition of 0.2% (v/v) formalin and incubation at 20°C for 4 days [284].

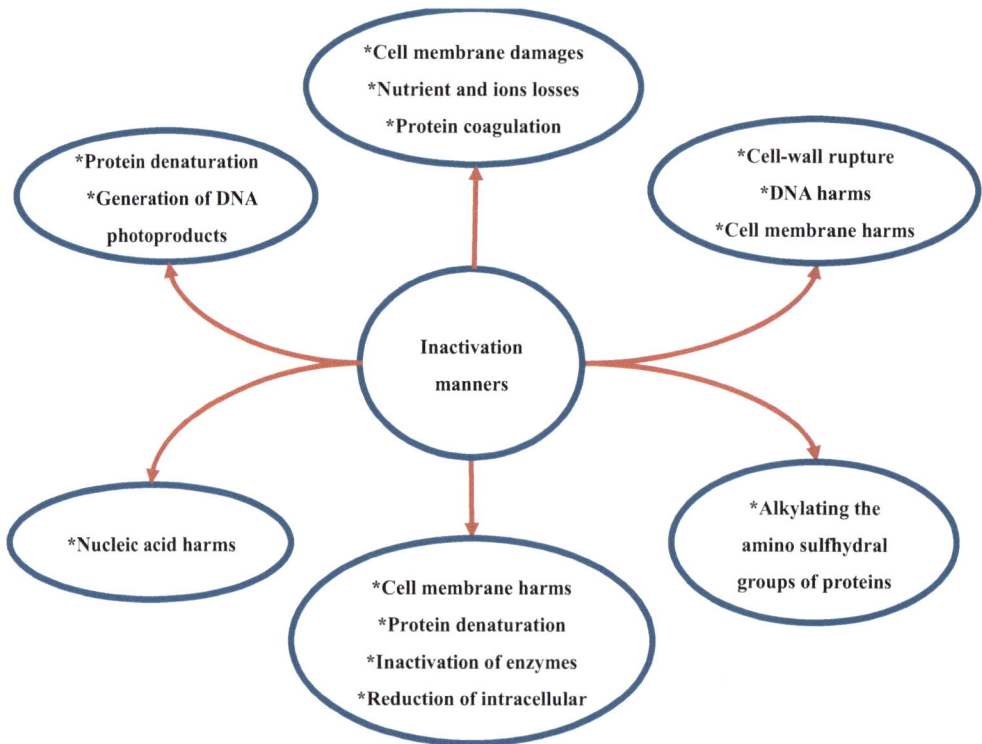

Fig. (5). The main mechanisms of conventional inactivation manners.

Sonication

The sonication manner, as a physical procedure, utilizes a sound wave with frequencies higher than the brink of human hearing to cleave intermolecular bonds [285]. In this technique, high pressure and temperature cause gas bubbles formation in liquid media that have the capability of exploring and generating intracellular cavitation, which in turn results in physicochemical alternations in cellular structures (disrupting cell membranes/cell wall, and DNA damage by Free Radical Species (FRS) generation) [286]. Moreover, the nature of the ultrasound waves, exposition time, microbial cells considered, and temperature determined the efficiency of this method [287, 288]. In a study [270], by using a sonifier cell disrupter (2 kHz, 40 min), researchers prepared a postbiotic from *L. plantarum* with satisfactory biological activity. Although there is a limited number of studies that highlight the inactivation of probiotic cells by the sonication method [282].

The Secondary Step in the Postbiotic Production Process

In most investigations, the fabrication of postbiotics was accomplished *via* deriving the cellular bioactive molecules from parent cells by centrifugation and ultrafiltration systems [255, 289, 290]. Nevertheless, the postbiotics collected may vary in terms of the quantities of peptides or proteins, bacteriocins, and organic acids about the media composition [290 - 293]. The laboratory production of postbiotics can be performed according to Foo *et al.*, [293], wherein the stock culture of the considered probiotic strain was resuscitated twice in the Man Rogosa Sharpe (MRS) broth and incubated for 48 and 24 h for each resuscitating period as a standing culture at 30°C. All the probiotic strains were grownup under anaerobic conditions at 30°C unless stated otherwise. Subsequently, the overnight culture was poured onto MRS agar and incubated anew till a single colony was created on the agar plate, which took up to 48 h. A single colony was selected, inoculated in MRS broth, and incubated overnight. An inoculum size of 1%-2% (v/v) from the overnight culture was anew moved and incubated overnight. Compounds were then gathered by centrifugation (12,000 ×*g* for 10 min at 4°C) to segregate the postbiotics from the parent cells. Gathered postbiotics were then filtered [292] previous to storage at 4°C until more use. About the following application, postbiotic components can also be prepared in powder form by spray drying technique [256]. Postbiotic components can also be formed in conditioned media [290], by incubation in a eukaryotic cell culture medium for the designated period. Probiotic cells segregated from food-based products may have various nutrient necessities to generate a wide range of postbiotic components. Leroy and Devust described that *Lactobacillus sakei* CTC 494 (as probiotic strain), isolated from fermented sausages, grow well in meat-based peptone; therefore the strains are well-regulated in the meat-like environment [294]. Ooi *et al.*, (2015), investigated the effects of different carbon and nitrogen sources on the bacteriocin-inhibitory activity of postbiotic metabolites generated *viaLactobacillus plantarum* I-UL4. They reported that the highest bacteriocin-inhibitory activity was attained at 1440 MAU/mL when 36.20 g/L of yeast extract and 20 g/L of glucose were added as the sole nitrogen and carbon sources respectively in the modified MRS medium [291]. On the other hand, the addition of peptone and meat extract diminutions the bacteriocin-inhibitory activity of the UL4 postbiotic components. Besides, it has been described that the addition of polysorbate 80 (Tween 80) significantly influenced the production of postbiotics (bacteriocin) by LAB [295, 296]. In this regard, polysorbate 80 can combine oleic acid with the cell membrane, which in turn possesses a significant increment in its liquidity to preserve the bacterial cells from harsh circumstances [297], and promoting nutrient uptake [298]. Parallel outcomes were stated by Tan *et al.*,

[292], whereby the polysorbate 80 addition to the reconstituted MRS media would significantly affect the proteinaceous postbiotic components generation *viaL. plantarum* I-UL4 [292]. In cytotoxicity investigation *versus* breast cancer cell lines, MCF-7 cells treated with the proteinaceous postbiotic components derived from *L. plantarum* I-UL4, cultivated in reconstituted MRS with polysorbate 80, revealed a higher percentage of apoptosis [292].

A Brief Discussion on the Extraction of Lipoteichoic Acids, Exopoly saccharides, and Peptidoglycan

Lipoteichoic Acids

Teichoic acids are negatively charged polymers bound to the cell wall of the majority of Gram-positive bacteria. They are composed of 30-40 subunits such as glycerol phosphate (Gro-P), ribitol phosphate (Rbo-P), or mannitol phosphate linked by a phosphodiester linkage. The main chain may also contain monosaccharide moieties (*e.g.* glucose, galactose, and rhamnose) and D-alanine. Depending on the binding to the cell wall, they can be dividing into two groups:1) wall teichoic acids (WTA), which are covalently bound to peptidoglycan, or 2) lipoteichoic acids (LTA), which are loosely anchoring in the cytoplasmic membrane. In the case of bacteria with G+C in their DNA higher than 50%, LTA is usually replacing by lipoglycans. They are made of linear or branched polysaccharides as a hydrophilic moiety, and they become charged by substitution with monoglycerol phosphate branches. Bifidobacterial teichoic acids belong to the less-known extracellular structures. Genome sequencing studies revealed that *Bifidobacterium* species contain the necessary genes needed to produce WTA and LTA. Colagiorgi *et al.* analysed genome of *B. bifidum* and found four homologs of *Bacillus subtilis gtaB* (UTP-glucose-1-phosphate uridylyltransferase), *ypfP* (glycosyltransferase_GTB_type), *pgcA* (phosphoglucomutase) and *ltaS* (phosphoglycerol transferase). However in bifidobacteria they coded glucose--phosphate thymidylyltransferase (BBPR_0078), UDPN-acetylglucosamine-N acetylmuramyl-(pentapeptide) pyrophosphoryl-undecaprenol-Nacetylglucosamine MurG (BBPR_0556*)*, phosphoglucomutase (BBPR_1512) and phosphoglycerol transferase (BBPR_1314). Interestingly, the transcription of genes responsible for LTA production isstimulating by environmental conditions. These may result in a difference in LTAs occurring in the intestine and *in vitro* cultivation [299].

Exopolysaccharides

Recently, exploiting safe probiotic compounds like exopolysaccharides (EPSs) (postbiotics) rather than probiotics, attracted great attention because of their various salutary effects. In line with this, in a recent study, it has been shown that

EPS derived from probiotic *L. paracasei*, results in apoptosis induction through down-regulation of the Akt1, mTOR, Jak-1, Bcl-2 mRNAs, and up-regulation of BAX, caspase-3, and caspase-8 genes in different colon cancer cell lines. Besides, the findings of the study demonstrated that the isolated EPS exerted insignificant cytotoxicity to normal cell lines [300].

Peptidoglycan

The cell wall of Gram-positive bacteria such as *Bifidobacterium* consists of most of peptidoglycan (PG), which can account for 30-70% of the cell wall surface. Its constitutive building blocks are *N*-acetylglucosamine (GlcNAc) and *N*-acetylmuramic acid (MurNAc) connected by β-1,4-Oglycosidic bonds that form a long polysaccharide chain [51]. It is cross-linked *via* a peptide chain to form a three-dimensional and rigid structure. In addition to the basic L- and D-amino acids, amino acids that are not typically founding in proteins can be part of the PG structure (*e.g.* L-ornithine). In the case of Gram-positive bacteria, two main types of PG designed as A and B are distinguished, which then sub-divide depending on the amino acid forming the bridge and the type of binding [301, 302].

QUALITY CONTROL: MAIN METHODS FOR IDENTIFICATION OF POSTBIOTICS

Metabolomics, as a powerful strategy, refers to the systematic identification and quantification of the small bio-molecules in complex biological systems, and so well appropriate for the recognition of various postbiotic components. A recent work by Kok *et al.* [303] applied chromatographic separation coupled with tandem mass spectrometry to describe the influence of antibiotic therapy on the metabolite index of rat urine specimens. In a parallel study, Antunes *et al.* [304] identified more than 2000 metabolite profiles in the case of rat feces specimens, and establish that a single high dose of streptomycin triggered noteworthy alterations in ~90% of these profiles. Until today, most investigations have applied an untargeted strategy to gain a complete profile of the changed metabolites. While this strategy has extensive application potential, it similarly has some disadvantages. Concurrent quantitative evaluation of a large number of metabolites applying mass spectrometry leftovers challenging due to the large dynamic variety of metabolites (up to 9 orders of value [305]) and sensibility restrictions. Without a prearranged set of targets, derivation protocol and mass spectrometry functioning factors cannot be appropriate for specific classes of metabolites to enhance sensibility. Unequivocal recognition of microbial metabolites could also present challenges if the sample comprises several ion parts that have the same mass signatures.

The development of targeted mass spectrometry [306] addresses some of these concerns, as a dedicated set of target metabolites can be improved for discovery and quantitation while still largely sampling the microbiota's biochemical variety. Furthermore, computational apparatuses have significant potential for assisting targeted mass spectrometry strategies and the identification of postbiotics. For instance, metabolic models of the gut microbiota could be applied to forecast the imaginable metabolites of dietary compounds and to recognize which of these metabolites most probably derived from the gut microbiota. In the last decade, genome-scale metabolic models (GEMs) have been developing that describe the gene-protein-reaction associations as well as metabolic potencies of specific tissues under different biological and disease circumstances [307]. The human models have also been applied as patterns to rebuilding GEMs for vital model organisms, remarkably the mouse [308, 309]. Currently, the main challenge in rebuilding GEMs is that the process is labor drastic, necessitating considerable manual endeavor to restore the information found in genome annotation databases, supposing that the species of attention have previously been sequenced and annotated in the first place [310 - 312].

A noteworthy work in modeling the metabolism of the gut microbiome is the effort by Greenblum *et al.*, who accumulated and evaluated a community-level metabolic network model to the discovery that there are topological diversities such as the connectivity of metabolic reactions as stated *via* their stoichiometry, amid normal, overweight, and IBS affected individuals [313]. More recently, Heinken employed flux balance analysis (as an extensively-applied method for analyzing metabolic networks) to investigate the metabolic interactions among an eminent representative human gut microbe, *Bacteroides thetaiotaomicron* (iAH991), and its murine host applying a GEM demonstrating the two species [314, 315].

In addition to restriction-based analyses such as flux balance analysis, an additional promising strategy for investigating community-level bio transformation applying metabolic network models is computational pathway analysis. In this regard, one example is Path-Miner, which forms bio transformation pathways of a user-determined starting metabolite to diminish the general energetic expense. Another algorithm, PathPred (as developed web-based server), employs templates of structural resemblances among the products of biochemical reactions and reactants to forecast potential degradation pathways. This algorithm is mainly valuable for artificial chemicals that are not common substrates of known enzymes [316]. Besides, Yousofshahi *et al.*, (2011), developed ProbPath, which combines flux balance analysis and graph analysis to recognize and rank potential synthesis routes for a user-determined target metabolite. The pathways identified in this study have formerly been confirming in the literature as viable, high-yield synthesis routes. Besides, this algorithm simplifies the design of unique and non-native synthesis routes through an efficacious exploring variety of biochemical transformations in nature [317]. In the case of forecasting postbiotic metabolism, a beneficial particularity of ProbPath is that it can electively recognize reactions that are non-indigenous to the host organism, therefore recognized metabolites that can form through one organism, such as an intestinal microbe but not through another such as human host. Currently, the most noteworthy restriction of ProbPath is the scarcity of properly constructed reaction databases for gut microbes. A promising *meta-metabolome* was established by Ibrahim and Anishetty, who assembled a small-scale metabolic network including 87 reactions of human gut microbiota (based on species belonging to the three predominant phyla namely *Firmicutes*, *Bacteroidetes*, and *Actinobacteria*) to investigate carbohydrate metabolism in the intestine [318]. It should be highlighted that prognostic approaches are only as valuable as the precision and comprehensiveness of the accessible genome annotation data, and the deficiency of awareness regarding the species comprising the microbiota has so far restricted in silico anticipation (Table **5**).

Table 5. Some important metabolome approaches applied for assessment and identification of postbiotic metabolites.

Item No.	Technologies
1	Mass-spectrometry
2	Gas chromatography
3	Pulsed-field gel electrophoresis
4	Nuclear magnetic resonance spectroscopy
5	Two-dimensional gel electrophoresis
6	Capillary electrophoresis with mass-spectrometry-based detection
7	High-efficiency high-resolution liquid chromatography with tandem high-resolution mass-selective detection
8	High-efficiency liquid chromatography with tandem high-resolution mass-selective detection with electrospray ionization
9	High-efficiency liquid chromatography with subsequently obtained mass spectrum in negative and positive modes of operation

CHAPTER 5

Bioactivity Perspectives and Health Benefits of Postbiotics

Abstract: Recent investigations have reported that the intestinal microbiome community possesses a significant health-promoting effect on the host physiology by the secretion of small biomolecules that exerts a unique ability to modulate the host cellular pathways. These small molecules act as a beneficial tool for host-microbial interactions and communication. Based on current evidence, postbiotics have the potency to be a safe and appropriate alternative to prevent side effects pertinent to probiotics besides the enforceable benefits such as treatments of some human complications. These beneficial effects are feasible through various mechanisms that are explained in related chapters. Some of the clinical advantages associated with postbiotics can refer to modulating the immune system, anti-diarrhea, anti-blood pressure activity, reducing blood cholesterol, anti-oxidant and anticancer activity, as well as suppressing cell proliferation. These properties indicate that postbiotics can improve the host's health circumstances, albeit with unknown mechanisms. Another substantial advantage of postbiotics returns to their desirable immune condition. In this case, there is no need to adsorb the trillions of live microorganisms. Besides, it is possible to impose the postbiotics in a controlled and standard way. However, the live microbes' functions depend on their interactions in the gut and their metabolical activities. Therefore, the compounds of specified bacteria may turn into a biological strategy as a complementary treatment of many important diseases. The main challenge in this respect is the scientific knowledge transformation to commercial applications, which constitute a bridge between science and industry.

Keywords: Aging, Atopic dermatitis, Anti-cancer therapy, Alcohol-induced liver diseases, Colitis, Diarrhea, Food allergy, Gut microbial community, Immunomodulation, Intestinal barrier, Inflammation, Lactose intolerance, Postbiotics, Probiotic, Tooth decay.

GUT MICROBIOME-BASED THERAPIES: A NEW APPROACH

All cavities and mucosal surfaces in the human body are occupied by a broad population of microorganisms [319]. The gut microbiota implicates in the host's multifunctional physiological processes, including immunity, nutritional and metabolic homeostasis, and neuronal activity [320]. Providing a stable niche for commensal microorganism colonization is a significant ability in the host. It ensures the stabilization of dietary nutrients. As technology progresses, in

Amin Abbasi, Elham Sheykhsaran & Hossein Samadi Kafil

metagenomics (genome sequencing) and gnotobiotics (germ-free mice usage), the remarkable involvement of human health-related microorganisms has become increasingly evident. Utilizing these apparatuses, we could expand our comprehension of the host and the microbiome interactions over the last decade. Related abnormalities in the gut microbiota composition and function are associated with the molecular etiology of multiple disorders. Several factors can lead to a loss of homeostatic function, including inflammation, infection, xenobiotics, hygiene, diet, altered host genetics, and microorganism diversity [137]. Consequently, efforts are ongoing to promoting health and modulating the human microbiome through device interventions. Due to the extensive role of microbiota in various gastrointestinal and non-gastrointestinal complications, it has become an interesting therapeutic target increasingly [138]. However, one of the most vital issues in microbiome research is determining cause-effect relationships and designing therapies based on the microbiome that can attain predictable benefits related to the host health and microbial community. A massive part of present microbiome-based therapeutics focuses on the microbiome-prokaryotic arm through the enforcing to modify the composition of the gut microbiota *via* the administration of exogenous live microbes. These approaches referred to probiotics term collectively, which has become a popular topic during the last decade. Nevertheless, there is still restricted evidence for supporting the efficacy of the probiotic. An appropriate alternative approach for probiotics is prebiotics. Besides, to live bacteria administration, prebiotics are considering consumed compounds to affect microbiome composition or function beneficially. Probiotics and prebiotics are considered as a comparatively non-specific approach for microbiome-based strategies, and more investigation is required to fully understand the effects of prebiotics on various bacterial species [18].

At present, a microbiome-based intervention is fecal microbiota transplantation (FMT) as a successful method approved by the FDA. FMT includes the whole microbial population transferring from a healthy donor to a recipient who suffered from some disorders to disease-associated microbiome replacement. FMT has been shown to include significant efficacy in *Clostridium difficile* infection treatment, which is conduct commonly followed by antibiotic therapy [321]. The utilizing of FMT for conditions of additional complications is investigating currently. Nonetheless, FMTs possibly are associated with the natural risk for the recipient, such as the pathobionts and undesirable interactions for the recipient with their current microbiome community. Because of the substantial variability of microbial community and individuals and the restricted long-term stabilization in foreign microbial configuration, opportunities are ample to alternative strategies that relevant to microbiome involvement in human health and understanding of it as a new mechanistic approach.

Recent investigations have reported that the intestinal microbiome community possesses a significant health-promoting effect on the host physiology by the secretion of small biomolecules that exerts a unique ability to modulate the host cellular pathways [322 - 325]. These small molecules act as a beneficial tool for the host's microbial interactions and communication. These pathways are including in target downstream signaling of the microbiome. Metabolite-based therapeutics, or "postbiotics," target the microbiome in terms of their downstream signaling pathways and play a vital role by moderating the side effects of an excess, insufficiency, or dysregulation of metabolites associated with these pathways. In comparison to targeting the composition of aberrant microbial, metabolites exogenous inhibition or administration has a potency for counteracting and correcting the negative impacts of dysbiosis (Fig. **6**). Primary instances of potential metabolite-based therapies that are existed in animal models of the human complications are involved short-chain fatty acids (SCFAs) with anti-inflammatory activity and in inflammatory bowel disease (IBD)-patients with altered properties [326 - 328]; flavonoids have been elucidated to have therapeutic effects on metabolic disorders [238]; and the organic acid taurine, recuperates the intestinal inflammation [208].

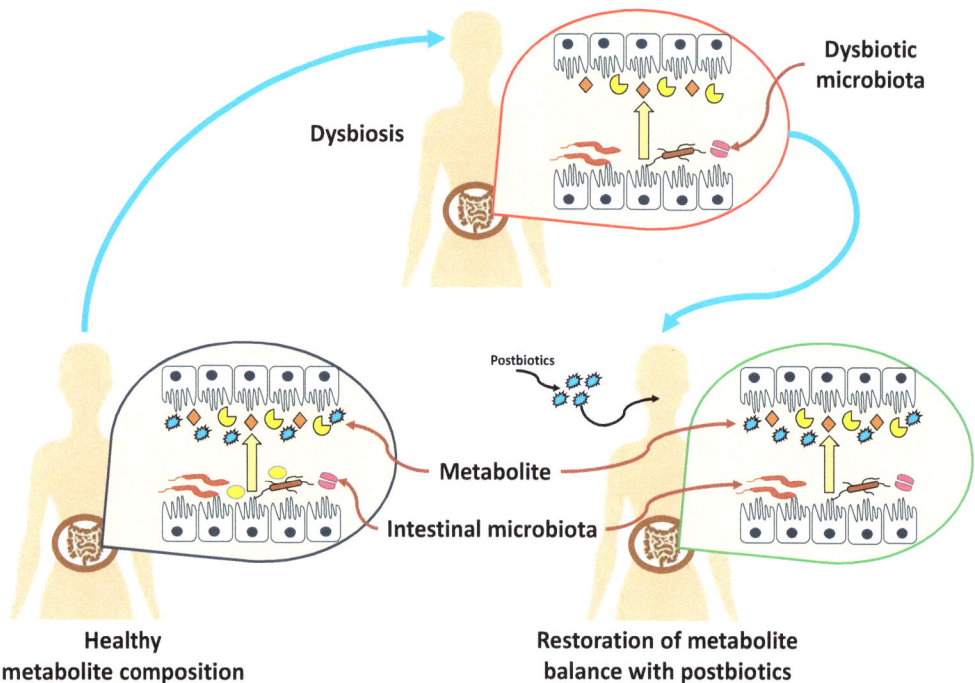

Fig. (6). The concept of metabolite-based therapeutics.

Under homeostatic circumstances, the gut microbiome generates, transforms, and degrades small molecules, which confer as actual means of communication in host-microbe connections and intensely influence human health status. Imbalances of the gut microbiome (dysbiosis) lead to later modifications in metabolite balances, which have been shown to have straight imports on host health in the context of various acute and chronic diseases. Metabolite/postbiotic-based therapeutics stimulate downstream signaling pathways of the gut microbiome and act *via* alleviating the undesirable effects of an abundance, shortage, or imbalances of metabolites involved in these pathways. For instance, the exogenous intake of postbiotics (pharmaceutical/food products) can consider the substantial therapy *versus* the consequences of dysbiosis.

Metabolite interventions are considered therapeutically interesting fields for many reasons. The small molecules have high concentrations physiologically, and therefore the toxic potential for them is low. In contrast, to live organism administration, the dosage of small molecules and administration routes follow the pharmacokinetics principles. Additionally, metabolites are found in the body on most sides and therefore are proper to various administration routes. Moreover, metabolites have enough stability in the systemic circulation. Hence, they are considered amenable to scalable modulation of their concentration. The metabolite-based therapeutics have a shorter half-life in comparison to the administration of live bacteria; therefore, repetitive dosing probably would be required for treating dysbiosis-related situations. Besides, microbiome-associated metabolite's impacts are pleiotropic and more cell type-specific. As such, more characterization of the full impacts of various metabolites is fundamental to comprehend the postbiotics' remarkable side effects. The microbiome-associated metabolite's functional impacts can widely be divided into two groups: integrated with the host's intracellular metabolism and receptor-mediated metabolite sensing (signaling molecules). In the former case, the microbiome functions act as an endocrine energy source to different tissues in the body [329]. In the case of, the latter microbiome-derived metabolites have the potency to be recognized directly through the host eukaryotic cells. Metabolites can initiate receptor-mediated signaling cascades and, therefore, stimulates the mediate cell-specific transcription, which can occur in the gastrointestinal tract locally or systemically. Such functions related to the signaling process have been recognizing for various metabolites and their interaction with the immune system, like the niacin, SCFAs, and indole derivatives [330]. A systematic effort is a need to identify microbiome-derived molecules and their mechanisms associated with the host senses and responses to them, which significantly reveals the precise mechanisms of metabolites on the host. Such a process by which the host can detect microbial elements is pattern recognition receptors (PRRs), including oligomerization domain-like receptors (NLRs) and nucleotide-binding. Microbial motifs recognition employing PRRs can initiate downstream signaling cascades, which lead to both tolerance and antimicrobial responses. A significant concern related to the approach of postbiotic is metabolites pleiotropic function. For instance, it has been demonstrating that SCFAs have many effects on human physiology, including intestinal integrity, regulation of appetite, metabolic control, and immune functions, which all these points are demonstrates to be related to health-improving [331]. Investigations of the dosage and administration route are critical for determining specific biological function mechanisms and their selective promotion. Even though the microbiome is proposing to be responsible for over half of all urinary and fecal metabolites, approximately a dozen metabolites presently have a well-characterized impact on the host, including receptors, target cells, physiological outcomes, and signaling pathways [332]. Systematic efforts are needed for a widening spectrum of well-characterized metabolites, utilizing defined readout systems and high-throughput technology. Finally, a comprehensive approach will allow us to investigate the principles of chemical design related to metabolite-host interactions. Can the classification of metabolites employing chemical structure enlighten us on how is metabolites bioactive function? Do metabolites derive from the microbiome cluster into a finite number of groups with the same functional relevance in the host? Will humans be able to anticipate the biological function of a metabolite according to biochemical relatedness to other metabolites ultimately? A fundamental insight is requiring for answering these questions to drivers of host-microbial coevolution.

PERSPECTIVES ON POSTBIOTICS BIOACTIVITY

Recently, a remarkable number of investigations employing *in vivo* (*e.g.*, hypertensive and obese rats) models and *in vitro* (*e.g.*, various cell lines) to survey important bioactivity and/or health impacts of different postbiotics, including cell wall components and intracellular metabolites either as isolated structures or mixtures, like the suspensions extracts [333].

In most instances, *Lactobacillus* and *Bifidobacterium* strains are postbiotics derivatives; however, *Faecalibacterium* and *Streptococcus* species have been shown as a postbiotics source as well [334]. It has been confirming that postbiotics supplementation decreases blood pressure it confers the capacity of antihypertensive for these components. The impacts of protective mechanism on the endothelial function have not been displaying; however, it can be as a result of modifications in the intestinal microbiota and its metabolic by-products; the restoration of the intestinal barrier function; and the impacts on inflammation, endotoxemia, and activity of renal sympathetic nerve [335].

Researches indicate that gut microbiota influence a broad range of functions in the gastrointestinal tract, such as immune system development, defending against pathogens, and inflammation [336]. Based on the advances in the postbiotics field, increasing data, mainly obtained by the *Lactobacilli* strains analysis, support much evidence that these useful impacts probably are depending on secreted-derived factors [337].

Immunomodulation is affected by retinoic acid-driven mucosal such as dendritic cells and following impacts on regulatory T-cells *in vitro* employing *L. reuteri* 17938, through the generating anti-inflammatory cytokine IL-10 [338]. In a related investigation, Sokol *et al.* (2008) reported that IL-8 increased levels in Caco-2 cells are exposing to the intracellular extracts and the *F. prausnitzii* supernatant fraction [339]. Furthermore, the data suggestions show the cell-free supernatant administration in TNBS-induced colitis case in a mice model, implemented an anti-inflammatory impact through the increasing IL-10, and decreasing IL-12, which demonstrated that secreted metabolites have the inducing ability and protective impacts. The research reported that the anti-inflammatory impact was related to a pathway independent from butyrate. Furthermore, the proposed mechanism was based on the activation of the NF-κB blockade; however, the involved and active molecules in this protective impact were not specified. More evidence has demonstrated that the *Lactobacillus paracasei* B21060 culture supernatant has protective healthy effects on tissue against the inflammation of invasive *Salmonella* in a human mucosa explant of the colon [340] and *Lactobacillus casei* DG culture supernatant can alleviate the inflammatory response in ileal and colonic mucosa cultures post-infectious bowel syndrome patients culture supernatant [337].

Besides, Cicenia *et al.* (2016) published that *Lactobacillus rhamnosus* GG supernatants obtained from various growth steps (middle and late exponential, stationary, and overnight) have protective effects on human colonic smooth muscle cells (HSMCs) against lipopolysaccharide (LPS)-induced myogenic destruction. The highest protective impacts were observed in the late stationary phase supernatants that reverted 84.1% of LPS-induced cell shortening and prevented 92.7% LPS-induced IL-6 secretion and 85.5% of acetylcholine-induced contraction [341].

Postbiotics have been explaining as an inhabitant agent for pathogenic bacteria against *Escherichia coli* E−30, *Salmonella enterica* S-1000, *Listeria monocytogenes* L-MS, and vancomycin-resistant *Enterococci* as pathogenic bacteria when employing cultures of cell-free supernatants obtained from *L. plantarum* RG11, RI11, RG14, TL1, UL4, and RS5 strains [342]. Moreover, *in vivo* and *in vitro* models with antioxidant activity exposed to specific exopolysaccharides (EPS) have been demonstrated as well. Xu, Shang, and Li

(2011) reported that EPS obtained from *Bifidobacterium animalis* RH demonstrating peroxidation of lipid *in vitro* inhibition and activity of radical scavenging (hydroxyl and superoxide radicals) [343]. Furthermore, Li *et al* . (2014) explained the extract of crude culture and purified EPS, derived from *Lactobacillus helveticus* MB2-1as an exhibiting agent and substantial scavenging capacity three kinds of free radicals and chelating ferrous ion capacity [344].

Specific instances of bacterial intracellular enzymes that have beneficial health benefits (*e.g.*, antioxidant) are including superoxide dismutase (SOD), glutathione peroxidase (GPx), NADH-peroxidase, and nicotinamide adenine dinucleotide (NADH)-oxidase [345, 346]. Additionally, some cell wall compounds are associated with immunomodulatory properties *in vitro* such as S-layer proteins, and lipoteichoic acids (LTA) [334]. Furthermore, many postbiotics demonstrate multiple bioactivities and can initiate multiple physiological pathways simultaneously. For instance, some cell wall compounds, like the LTA, have a broad range of bioactivities such as antitumor, antioxidant, and immunomodulatory capacities [347, 348]. Besides, sterol-like compounds in the microbial membrane have received more attention such as plasmalogens as endogenous antioxidants that confer resistance to H_2O_2-induced oxidative stress in many strains of *Bifidobacterium* [349, 350].

Based on other researches, gut microbiota produced-SCFAs serve as signaling molecules to the regulation improvement of glucose homeostasis, metabolism of lipid, and insulin sensitivity, utilizing the activation of the receptor-like the G protein-coupled receptors (GPRs), therefore, they contribute to the energy balance regulation and maintaining metabolic homeostasis [351, 352]. Specific SCFAs (*e.g.* acetate, butyrate, and propionate) have been proving to play a role in plasma cholesterol homeostasis in humans and rodents [353].

The postbiotics hepatic-protective role has been previously explaining. Suspension of Cell lysate from *Lactobacillus fermentum* BGHV110 decreases hepatotoxicity induced by acetaminophen in HepG2 cells through the autophagy activation in HepG2 cells employing the PINK1 signaling pathway [289]. In a related investigation, Sharma *et al.* (2011) published the hepatic-protective impact of intracellular content of *Lactobacillus acidophilus* MTCC447 and *Enterococcus lactis* IITRHR1 against hepatotoxicity induced by acetaminophen in a cultured rat hepatocytes model. Besides, the authors discovered the potency of postbiotics for restoring the level of glutathione and reducing the role of oxidative stress biomarkers levels [354, 355].

Besides, postbiotics presumably are generated by yeast metabolic activity. Canocini *et al.* (2011) declared that *Saccharomyces boulardii* culture supernatants promote the wound healing process and migration of epithelial cells through the α2β1 integrin collagen receptors activation employing *in vitro* models. Furthermore, the authors found that daily oral administration of these culture supernatant to mice during 7 days recuperate migration of enterocytes in small intestinal tissues along the crypt-villus axis [355]. This information recommended that these supernatants can be recuperated the intestinal epithelium repairing after injuries (restitution of intestine) and exert a potential therapeutic effect in a wide variety of gastrointestinal complications.

Discovering postbiotics bioactive properties recommend that these components presumably contribute to the host health-improving through providing appropriate specific physiological impacts, employing the combined impacts of postbiotics, the live microorganism, and other biological metabolites. This synergism probably results in over-effective protective qualities [356].

The protective impacts of postbiotics can be manifested by mimicry components of the useful and therapeutic impacts of probiotics, although the action mechanisms probably are different. For example, probiotic bacteria's hypocholesterolemic mechanisms are included in the inhibition of intestinal cholesterol absorption and/or the prevention of bile acid reabsorption [357]. Additionally, postbiotics have an activating impact on the receptor activated by the peroxisome proliferator, it is considered as a causative agent for fatty acid β-oxidation to decreasing triglycerides [358]. Besides, postbiotics activate the oligomerization domain-containing protein 1 binding to nucleotide for inducing adipocyte's cell-autonomous lipolysis [359], to reduce the hepatic 3-hydroxy-3-methyl glutaryl-CoA synthase (HMGCS) enzyme activity and 3-hydroxy-3-methyl glutaryl-CoA reductase (HMGCR), and to elevate the protein kinase activated by AMP in muscle tissue and liver [353], therefore, leads to improving the dyslipidemia control and lipid metabolism. Moreover, it has been elucidating that postbiotics based on muramyl dipeptide probably decrease the inflammation of adipose and intolerance of glucose through a nucleotide-binding oligomerization domain-containing protein 2 and by the transcription factor IRF4 activation in obese mice [355]. Furthermore, this postbiotic decreases the insulin resistance in hepatic cells in low-level endotoxemia and obesity.

Postbiotics have been confirming as an anti-proliferative specific compound against the cancerous cells in the colon, most likely associated with the pro-apoptotic cell death pathways activation utilizing immune response regulation [360]. It has been shown that obtained *Lactobacillus* strains- postbiotics presumably reduce the inhibition activity of metalloproteinase-9 in colon cancer invasion [361]. To demonstrate the active compound account for this impact, the postbiotic (cell-free supernatant) was fractionated according to molecular weight ranges; it was elucidated that the inhibitory fraction activity corresponded to the 50–100 kDa and >100 kDa compounds, proposing that the inhibitory components probably act as a macromolecule such as nucleic acids, protein, or polysaccharides.

Some researchers [362 - 364] reported that lactic acid bacteria-derived cell-free extracts presumably show remarkably more antioxidant capacity compared to whole-cell cultures; it suggests that the antioxidant capacity is associated with enzymatic and non-enzymatic intracellular antioxidants. Additionally, *Bifidobacterium* infantis, *B. adolescentis* , *B. breve* , and *B. longum* can degrade hydrogen peroxide through the NADH peroxidase production [365]. Glutathione reductase and glutathione peroxidase are considering two applicable antioxidant enzymes that have protective effects on cells against oxidative destruction through the scavenging reactive oxygen species (ROS). However, this antioxidant enzyme activity is not able to be positively associated with all strains. This point demonstrates that other components probably are involved in the antioxidant effect [345]. It is believed that *Lactobacillus* different strains intracellular fraction have positive antioxidant capacity related to the cellular content of decreased glutathione, as a significant non-enzymatic antioxidant that plays an important role in the maintenance of intracellular redox state [366]. The scavenging properties of ROS and reactive nitrogen species are associated with the antioxidant activity of such non-enzymatic postbiotic [367].

Besides, antioxidant activity is a property of exopolysaccharides [368]. According to some investigations, this activity is associated with raised contents of uronic acid. Li *et al.* [344] suggested that uronic acid has a crucial role in the antioxidant activity of polysaccharides derived from *B. animalis* RH and *L. helveticus* MB2-1. Also, they revealed that there is a polysaccharide derived from *L. helveticus* MB2-1, with a huge proportion of negative charged uronic acid, which generated more chelating capacity ferrous ion. Ferrous ions play a role in the free radicals generated by the Fenton and Haber-Weiss reactions, which produce reactive hydroxyl radicals. Based on the reports, there is a direct association between the radical scavenging capacity of tea polysaccharides and uronic acid content [369].

It has been recommending that postbiotics anti-inflammatory and immunomodulatory abilities are mediating through the induction and inhibition of the immune systems in different animal models. It has been demonstrated that postbiotics have regulatory effects on cytokine response production and inhibition of the Th1 pathway [370]. The postbiotics antimicrobial activity presumably is associated with the several known and unknown antimicrobial components present, generally including enzymes, small molecules, bacteriocins, and organic acids, which demonstrate bactericidal or bacteriostatic properties against the

Gram-negative and Gram-positive bacteria [342].

García-Carrizo *et al.*, (2019), used mild calorie restriction-rats as a model of metabolic malprogramming consisting of the progeny during their pregnancy, both under an obesogenic (high-sucrose) and diet control, High-esterified pectin (HEP) supplement, in part with *in vitro* investigations in primary cultured white and brown adipocytes treated with the acetate includes postbiotic. The researchers proposed that supplementation of chronic HEP stimulates brown and white adipose tissue's markers thermogenic ability, with a reduction in energy efficiency, and weight gain prevention within an obesogenic diet. HEP increases the number of useful bacteria in the intestine and acetate peripheral levels. Furthermore, acetate *in vitro* can develop the production of adipokine, and elevate the thermogenic ability and browning in brown and white adipocytes, respectively, which are considered as a protection mechanism to obtain weight gain demonstrated *in vivo*. It had been concluded that acetate and HEP stand out as prebiotic/postbiotic active components capable of modulating both brownings and protect against obesity and brown-adipocyte metabolism [371].

Riaz Rajoka *et al.*, (2019), studied the three *Lactobacillus rhamnosus* strains SHA111, SHA112, and SHA113 anticancer activity, the isolates were obtained from human breast milk. In this investigation the liquid culture cell-free supernatant of the three strains exhibited significant antioxidant activity against superoxide anion radicals, DPPH free radicals, and hydroxyl radicals; additionally, remarkable anticancer activity was observed on cervix cancer cells (HeLa) through the cytotoxicity and apoptosis induction. They performed RT-qPCR and western blot analysis to indicating the apoptosis induction responses that were achieved by up-regulation of BAX, BAD, Caspase3, Caspase8, Caspase9, and down-regulation of HeLa cells' BCL-2 genes. These results recommend that the mentioned strains of postbiotics have remarkable anticancer capability [372]. All mentioned properties recommend that postbiotics presumably lead to the host's health status improvement through providing proper and specific physiological impacts, even though, the precise mechanisms are not well-understood.

PERSPECTIVES ON THE HEALTH BENEFITS OF POSTBIOTICS

According to the existing evidence, postbiotics have included some beneficial health effects such, as probiotics. However, the consumption probiotics is not always harmless. Several investigations report the inflammatory responses following the probiotics intake [373, 374]. Therefore, postbiotics have the potency to be a safe and insure alternative to prevent side effects pertinent to probiotics besides the functional benefits such as treating some human complications. These beneficial effects are feasible through various mechanisms that are explaining complete in related chapters. Some clinical advantages associated with postbiotics are modulation of the immune system, anti-diarrhea, anti-blood pressure activity, reduce blood cholesterol, anti-oxidant activity, and suppresses cell proliferation [87]. These properties indicate that postbiotics can improve the host health circumstances even though with unknown mechanisms. Another important advantage of postbiotics returns to their desirable immune circumstances, in this case, there is no need to adsorb the trillions of live microorganisms. Besides, it is possible to impose the postbiotics in a controlled and standard way. However, the live microbes' functions depend on their interactions in the gut and metabolically activities-related strains [86]. Therefore, the compounds of selective and certain bacteria may turn into a biological strategy as a complementary treatment of many important diseases. The main challenge in this respect is the scientific knowledge transformation to commercial applications, which constitute a bridge between science and industry. Currently, secreted metabolites of beneficial bacteria are termed as products with potential drug applications in the prevention and treatment of diseases. For instance, Colibiogen as a derived product from Escherichia coli culture has contained some compounds such as amino acid, peptide, polysaccharide, and fatty acids with preventative properties to resistant and susceptible *Salmonella* strains to antibiotics *in vitro*. Also, Colibiogen has significant efficiency in intestinal colitis treatment and alleviating skin ulcers in polymorphous light eruptions-patients. It has been reporting that a lysis form of the probiotic cell has to include hyaluronic acid, sphingomyelinase, lipoteichoic acid, exopolysaccharide, peptidoglycan, lactic acid, and acetic acid that constitute extensive biological activities with beneficial effects on eczema, dermatitis, and protect from ultraviolet light [86, 282]. The effects of postbiotics on human complications will be discussed in detail in the next stories.

The Effect of Postbiotics in the Growth Inhibition of the Pathogenic Microbes

Postbiotics are similar to probiotics can protect their hosts from infections caused by pathogenic microbes. Research has shown that heat-treated *Bacillus subtilis* and *Lactobacillus delbrueckii* can lead to an increase in respiratory burst and leukocyte peroxidase levels, which can eventually lead to the elimination of pathogenic microbes [375]. The postbiotics derived from heat-inactivated *Lactobacillus plantarum* can protect the host against systemic infection caused by *Salmonella enterica*. It seems that postbiotics can inhibit the invasion and attachment of pathogenic bacteria to epithelial cells [133]. Another study looked at the effect of postbiotics on inhibiting the growth of viruses and found that the consumption of heat-inactivated *Lactobacillus* reduces the risk of mice becoming infected with the flu H1N1 virus by increasing immune responses in the gut, respiratory tract and increasing interferon-beta titers [376, 377]. Also, feeding the viable and non-viable form of *Lactobacillus acidophilus* to mice infected with the flu H1N1 virus significantly increases the elimination of the virus as a result of the activity of natural killer cells [378]. It has also recently been demonstrated that the oral use of heat-inactivated *Lactobacillus lactis* can induce antiviral reactions in healthy individuals against the influenza virus (A/H3N2, A/H1N1) [379]. Postbiotics have also been used to prevent diseases in other organisms, such as aquatic animals. In one study, the effect of heat-inactivated *Lactobacillus plantarum* on the safety parameters of a freshwater shrimp species was investigated. It was found that postbiotics can detect by pathogen-associated molecular pattern receptors or hemocytes (substitutes for normal immune cells in crustaceans), which in turn significantly reduces the shrimp mortality caused by pathogenic bacteria such as *Aeromonas hydrophila* [106].

The Effect of Postbiotics in the Immunomodulation

Commensal microbes and innocuous dietary antigens target the mucosal immune system continuously in the intestine. In addition to the significant effect on metabolic function and intestinal homeostasis, this local microbial population has a remarkable role in form the response of immune cells for their functional role in particular tissues. For example, gut epithelial cells affect the intestinal dendritic cells (DC) related response, which influences subsequent responses of T cells. Some epithelial cells-produced substances including indoleamine 2,3-dioxygenase and thymic stromal lymphopoietin pose a tolerogenic phenotype in DC [380]. Epithelial cells have the ability to vitamin A metabolize into retinoic acid (RA) as well. Of the most important pleiotropic impacts, RA has been demonstrated to advance the precursor of CD103+ DC and pre-DC migration into the small intestine and inducing expression of CD103+ in monocyte-derived (Mo-) DC *in vitro*. Coculturing T cells with RA-DC has inducing effects on the gut homing markers CCR9 and α4β7 upregulation, and incorporator production of IL10 in T cells, however, the RA-DC response to intestine microbes has not yet been assessed *in vitro*. Absorption and digestion of foods and unhealthy and/or useless waste products omission like the pathogenic organisms and antigens are the main roles of the gastrointestinal tract [381]. Homeostasis of the gastrointestinal tract is mainly unique and preserved through the functions of mucosal immune cells such as Th1, Th2, Th17, and regulatory T (Treg) cells, fundamental functions of Gut-associated Lymphoid Tissues (GALT), antimicrobial peptides like the secretory IgA, defensins, and gut commensal microbes and their by-products (postbiotics). Of the most important roles in GALT is immune tolerance induction as a basic factor in preserve mucosal homeostasis because of the major numbers of foreign components, especially food proteins, that antigen-presenting cells (APCs) of the intestinal mucosa collision [382].

Modulation of the Gut Microbiota: An Effect of Postbiotics

The gut microbiota implements a basic role in the nutritional, metabolic, physiological, and immunological functions in the human body as significant metabolic activities through utilizing diet energy. Probiotics can promote the balance of gut microbiota [383]. *Lactococcus lactis* ssp. *lactis* G50 (heat-inactivated, lyophilized, and added in the diet at 0,5 g/Kg) as the postbiotic, ameliorate the gut microbiota in accelerated senescence- mice, it has preventative activity on the noxious intestinal bacteria's growth. G50 prevents the intestinal H_2S-producing bacteria's growth. However, its mechanism is not clear complete. Therefore, it is elemental to clear if G50 as a postbiotic adheres to gut cells or has co-aggregates interaction with pathogens [384].

The Impact of Postbiotics in the Recuperation of Intestinal Injuries

The gut is a co-exist environment where microorganisms and hosts have an equilibrium condition. The interactions of microbiota in the host provide health usages to the former. Useful microorganisms, including probiotics, have been employing to promote intestinal damages. *L. brevis* SBC8803 (heat-inactivated and suspended in PBS) as a postbiotic decreases the intestinal injuries and inflammation in mice that suffer from dextran sodium sulfate-induced colitis in comparison to the untreated mice. SBC8803 improves the barrier function of the gut epithelium through the heat shock protein stimulation. Investigations show that inflammation of the intestine has been recuperated by pro-inflammatory cytokines regulation and cell differentiation [385].

The Impact of Postbiotics in Intestinal Barrier Preservation and Reduction of Bacterial Translocation

The gut barrier is an important defense mechanism utilizing in maintaining gut integrity and protecting the organism from the environment [386]. Dysfunction of the gut barrier allows the antigens (bacteria and their toxins) to enter as a bacterial translocation [387]. Probiotics have maintaining use in the gut barrier and decrease bacterial translocation. Postbiotics like the *Sac. boulardii* (heat-inactivated and saline- suspended at 109 CFU/mL) preserves the mice's gut barrier by maintaining gut permeability and decreasing bacterial translocation. It seems that these useful impacts are depending on the postbiotics structural components, presumably the cell wall pf the yeast. Hence, the mechanism affects the cell structure more in comparison to the metabolism [388]. Yogurt contains postbiotics (*S. thermophilus, L. bulgaricus,* and *L. acidophilus* heat-inactivated,

1×10^9 cells/mL) was remarkably useful in disruption preventing the process of the intestinal epithelial barrier function in human gut Caco-2 cells. The capable mechanism affects the activation and production of subsequent nitric oxide (NO) stimulated by pro-inflammatory cytokines [389].

The Postbiotics Effects on the Treatment of Diarrhea

Diarrhea is considered a common gastrointestinal complication related to a raised bowel movement, consistency of the feces modifications, abdominal pain, distension, and a sensation of incomplete evacuation. Some probiotics have been demonstrating to be beneficial for diarrhea treatment. Postbiotic capsules have contained 5 billion cells that are killing with heat, and lyophilized *L. acidophilus* LB (French Lacteol Fort) has been utilizing in chronic diarrhea treatment in humans recuperates the symptoms like abdominal pain, feces consistency, distension, and the sensation of incomplete evacuation [390]. Lacteol Fort has some beneficial usages in the treatment of viral or bacterial diarrhea in children, decreasing the disease duration, and promoting feces consistency [391]. The postbiotics recuperate the symptoms of irritable bowel syndrome- patients, with a predominance of diarrhea, swelling, reducing the pain, and the score for health-related quality of life (HRQOL), which is proportional inversely to the life quality. Also, postbiotics decrease many weekly evacuations and the fecal incontinence rate. It seems that the Lacteol action mode is associated with the *L. acidophilus* LB ability to line the colic mucous, protecting it from pathogen adhesion and invasion [392]. Furthermore, the fermented milk administration, which has contained heat-inactivated *L. gasseri* CP2305 (1×10^{10} cells/container), for three weeks, leads to defecation and stool characteristics improvements (color tone). Therefore, this postbiotic regulates intestinal function in a tendency toward constipation- patients [392].

The Impact of Postbiotics in Colitis Treatment

The inflammatory intestinal disorder is considered a chronic inflammatory complication that influences the GIT and has consisted of two important forms: Crohn's disease and ulcerative colitis [393]. Some postbiotics have been demonstrated to include useful impacts on colitis prevention or development . *B. breve* and *B. Bifidum* postbiotics (lyophilized and heat-inactivated) manifest an anti-inflammatory impact on peripheral blood mononuclear cells (PBMNC) derived from ulcerative colitis-patients. The postbiotics administration stimulates the interleukin 10 (IL-10) production in the PBMNC of ulcerative colitis-patients and prevents the IL-8 secretion in epithelial cells. IL-10 as an anti-inflammatory cytokine has a crucial role in the inflammatory responses controlling. IL-8 is pertinent to the inflammation of ulcerative colitis patients. These regulatory properties conducted by *B. breve* and *B. bifidum* postbiotics on the ILs contribute to control gut inflammation, providing a protective impact on ulcerative colitis-patients [394]. Besides, *L. brevis* SBC8803 postbiotics (lyophilized and heat-inactivated) promotes the gut destructions in colitis-suffering mice induced by dextran sodium sulfite (DSS) *via* promoting the gut barrier [385].

The Effect of Postbiotics on the Digestive System Functions

The gut commensal microbiota plays a key role in the body's metabolic, nutritional, physiological, and immunological processes [395]. Table **6** summarizes the positive role of postbiotics in modulating the intestinal microbial population, improving intestinal lesions, treating diarrhea, and reducing lactose intolerance. Maintenance of the epithelial barrier integrity and the improvement of its functions depend on postbiotic components application as a novel approach. In this case, postbiotics basic mechanisms have been indicated *in vivo* and *in vitro* investigations as follow: 1) genes stimulation of tight-junctions of encoding constituents, 2) reassembly of protein through transcription factors triggering including SP1, 3, and STAT, 3) improve the resistance of colonic cells transepithelial electricity in human (Caco-2, T84), rat (cdx2-IEC) and porcine (IPEC-J2) small intestine cells, 4) Antimicrobial Peptides (AMPs) generation through the gut Epithelial Cells, and 5) epithelial barrier function reestablishment in inflammatory conditions like the Inflammatory Bowel Diseases (IBD). Moreover, allergy-protective commensal bacteria colonization (*e.g.* Clostridia) and SCFA as their metabolites motivate ILC3s in the colonic Lamina Propria (LP) to generate IL-22 as the barrier-protective cytokine. The IL-22 generation promotes the efficacy of epithelial barrier through the discharge of mucus adjusting using goblet cells and AMPs production by Paneth cell. IL-22-conducts functional responses and decreases f dietary antigens' accessibility to the systemic circulation in the host and appreciably decreases allergic sensitization [396].

The Role of Postbiotics in the Reduction of Lactose Intolerance

Lactose intolerance is a common gastrointestinal disorder. The prevalence in Asia is estimating at 50%, and in some Asian countries, it is as high as 100% [400]. Lactose intolerance can detect *via* the symptoms of bloating, swelling, nausea, vomiting, abdominal pain, abdominal distention, and diarrhea after lactose consumption, as well as by performing a Hydrogen breath test (HBT). A study conducted by Rampengan *et al.* examined the effect of prescribing sachets containing postbiotic compounds (Dialac) in children with lactose intolerance. In this study, the HBT test was applied, and a scale of more than 20 ppm was considered lactose intolerance. The result showed a significant reduction in the HBT scale of the patients. So, they are concluded that postbiotic sachets can reduce the symptoms of the disease and improve the health status of the affected children [401]. Therefore postbiotics can enter the stage of industrial production to promote community health.

Table 6. The effect of postbiotics on gastrointestinal disorders.

Gastrointestinal Disorder	Etiology	Postbiotic Functions	References
Disorders in the composition of the gut microbial	The gut microbial population can be altered by the overuse of antibiotics and some infections, which in turn, can lead to other illnesses.	Probiotic bacteria can modulate the population of the intestinal microbiome and through interaction with them to facilitate the production of some metabolites. Inactivated *Lactobacillus gasseri* increase *Clostridium* metabolites (type IV), also this bacteria can produce short-chain fatty acids such as acetate.	[397]
Intestinal ulcers	Inflammation and damage to intestinal tissue occur as a result of infection or drug use. Crohn's and ulcerative colitis are inflammatory bowel diseases.	The consumption of postbiotics can contributes to improving colitis by inducing heat shock proteins and regulating the secretion of (TNF-α) and some interleukins.	[385, 394]
Irritable bowel syndrome	A chronic disease that is associated with abdominal pain, discomfort, bloating, diarrhea, and/or constipation.	Inactivated *Lactobacillus gasseri* leads to a reduction in the inflammation responses in chronic diseases such as irritable bowel syndrome.	[339, 398]
Diarrhea	Bacterial and viral infections, antibiotics, and other factors can cause excessive fluid outflow in the form of diarrhea.	Inactivated *Lactobacillus casei* reduces the incidence of diarrhea in infants.	[91]
Lactose intolerance	The deficiency of lactase enzyme causes indigestion of dietary lactose and the emergence of lactose intolerance. Lactose fermentation by the intestinal flora produces large amounts of gas and acid that eventually causes gastrointestinal complications.	The consumption of postbiotics can reduce the symptoms of lactose intolerance in children.	[399]

The Impact of Postbiotics on the Alcohol-Induced Liver Diseases Improvement

The elevated incidence rates of alcohol-induced complications of the liver in different countries all over the world are relating to alcoholic beverages overconsumption. Alcohol chronic consumption can result in a fatty liver situation characterized by cholesterol and triglycerides accumulation [402]. A significant interaction between the gut and liver is similar to the alcohol, which can stimulate the alterations in the gut microbiota and permeability of the intestine and accelerate the progression to liver complications [403]. Investigations have demonstrated the probiotic's important role in pathogenesis control in alcohol-induced liver complications cases. Postbiotic derived from *L. brevis* SBC8803 (lyophilized, heat-inactivated, and added in the diet at 1.45×10^9 CFU/mg) was administered to alcohol-feeding mice, and the results showed an ability to improving the alcohol-induced liver complications. Hence, this point can consider as a promising agent for preventing and alleviate the situation. These postbiotics can hinder the elevated levels of alanine aminotransferase (ALT) and aspartate aminotransferase (AST) in the serum, and liver's total cholesterol and triglycerides in alcohol consumption cases. The role of ALT and AST enzymes are shown in the hepatocytes, and destructed hepatocytes, their main effect has been conducted by the migration into the blood. *L. brevis* SBC8803 postbiotics supplementation prevents the RNAm's over-expression in the tumor necrosis factor-α (TNF-α), the regulation of sterol element-binding protein 1 (SREBP-1), SREBP-2 in the liver and elevates the heat shock protein 25 (Hsp25) expression in the small intestine. The main role of TNF-α as an inflammatory cytokine is in liver pathogenesis. Reducing TNF-α expression is presumably due to the prevention of its production in the liver. SREBP-1 and SREBP-2 serve as regulatory agents in the involved genes in the transcription and synthesis of triglycerides and cholesterol, respectively. A decreasing rate in the SREBPs expression contributes to triglycerides and cholesterol reduction in the liver. Hsps confer protection on the cells in thermal, oxidative, and inflammatory stress conditions. A raised rate in Hsp25 in the epithelial cells enforces the epithelial barrier against destruction and preserving the barrier function. It seems that *L. brevis* promotes induced damages in the liver and the fatty liver situation through the decreasing SREBPs and TNF-α expressions [402].

The Postbiotics Impact on the Modulation of Inflammation

A complex reaction of the immune system is inflammation, which involves plasma proteins as well as activation and accumulation of leukocytes regarding the infection, cell damage, or toxins exposition. When equilibrated, inflammation implemented a protective function, control the infection, and inducing tissue repair. When the complication is not under control, it has the ability to tissues damage [388]. Probiotics have to decrease inflammation, for example, postbiotics and probiotics derived from *L. rhamnosus* GG can decrease the inflammatory response stimulated by lipopolysaccharides in rats. The probiotics can decrease pro-inflammatory mediators and elevate the anti-inflammatory mediators as well. Diluted in rat milk substitute-postbiotics GG or RMS (10^8 CFU/L) was demonstrated to have efficiency as the probiotic strain in the inflammation lipopolysaccharides-stimulated modulation. It seems that the postbiotic *L. rhamnosus* GG provided modulation is applied because of the cell components like the peptidoglycan and cell wall, and lipoteichoic acid, however, further investigations are needed for elucidating the involved exact mechanism [404]. Besides, postbiotics and probiotics derived from *L. rhamnosus* GG (UV-inactivated and culture media- suspended without antibiotics at 10^{11} CFU/L) were able to modulate the flagellin-induced inflammation in Caco-2 intestinal epithelial cells. IL-8 as the pro-inflammatory cytokine was utilized for measuring the inflammation. The postbiotics and probiotics from *L. rhamnosus* GG decrease the IL-8 production in the gut epithelium and modulating the inflammation [405].

The Effect of Postbiotics in the Growth Inhibition of the Cancer Cells

Anti-tumor properties are the main feature of probiotic bacteria that have attracted a lot of attention [406]. The outcomes of recent studies demonstrated that prob-iotics possess a significant reducing effect on some side-effects of conventional cancer therapies on the hosts [407]. Most studies have to focus on probiotics; but, the inactivated form effects of these bacteria have recently been investigating. Evidence from clinical studies confirms the positive effect of postbiotics in this field. In this regard, in a randomized clinical trial study, patients were divided into two groups, the first group receiving only placebo and the second group taking postbiotic supplements in addition to placebo. The results of the study showed a significant reduction in the severity of diarrhea, abdominal pain, vomiting, inflammation of the oral mucosa, atrophy, skin lesions, immune and cardiovascular disorders in the second group compared to the first group [408]. Some important mechanisms involved in the biological function of postbiotics in improving cancer therapies include: reducing cell viability, improving immune responses, inhibiting carcinogens and mutagenic agents, activating cell death pathways, reducing microbial invasion and its caused inflammation, increasing apoptosis rate in comparison to necrosis, reducing the activity of metalloproteinase-9, and offering anti-proliferative properties against cancerous cells [409]. Therefore, postbiotics due to their biological roles in improving conventional cancer therapies and reducing their possible adverse effects can be used in the form of pharmaceutical or food delivery systems along with other therapies for the prevention and treatment of cancer.

The Role of Postbiotics in the Improvement of Food Allergy

Food allergy is recognized as the most common immune disorder, and it can be derived from a breakdown of immune tolerance. Food allergy has been considered as a world health risk that influences the quality of life of patients, particularly in developed countries [87]. In the last two decades, the prevalence of clinical symptoms associated with a food allergy, especially in developed countries, has increased significantly, which is also economically important [410]. According to the results of studies on a wide range of foods, more than one hundred and seventy types of food were associated with a food allergy, so that the most important of these are fishery products such as fish and shellfish, dairy products such as milk, wheat, soy, eggs, nuts, and seeds [411]. The studies that focused on examining the role of the gut microbiota in promoting the host's health status, showed a direct and complex relationship between the composition of the gut microbiota and the function of the immune system. In this regard, in a situation that beneficial microbiota (probiotics) are predominant in the intestinal environment modulate the symptoms of food allergy *via* direct contact to the epithelial and immune cells [412]. According to the results of clinical trials, postbiotic components such as short-chain fatty acids (butyrate) play a significant role in reducing food allergy symptoms in the host. These postbiotics exert inductive reactions with the host's immune cells and reduce the sensitivity of the host against harmless antigens [413]. Short-chain fatty acids derived from *Lactobacillus* and *Bifidobacterium* species are important sources of energy for intestinal cells, besides, their attached to G-protein-coupled receptors (GPCRs) (located at the top of the colonocytes, enterocytes, and immune cells) and stimulates epithelial dendritic cells and macrophages to produce interleukin 10 (IL-10). On the other hand, they mediate the development of regulatory T lymphocytes (Tregs) in mesenteric lymph nodes, which ultimately lead to inhibition of inflammatory responses and food allergy [410, 414]. Due to the positive effects of postbiotics in establishing a coherent relationship with the immune system and establishing appropriate immune responses to reduce host sensitivity to the presence of certain antigenic factors as well as reducing inflammatory symptoms, they are considered as a novel strategy in improving food allergy [87].

The Effect of Postbiotics in the Reduction of Cholesterol Level

According to the Heart, Lung, and Blood Institute, a heart attack is one of the leading causes of death in the United States. Several factors can contribute to this problem, but one of the most important is to increase blood cholesterol levels. *Lactobacillus acidophilus* can sediment cholesterol in its cellular coating [415]. This phenomenon has also been observed in heat-inactivated bacteria such as

Lactococcus lactis, which is due to the absorption of cholesterol by cell-wall compounds. However, since live bacteria also trap some cholesterol in their cellular structures, the amount of cholesterol harvested in cases where live bacteria are using is up to three times higher [416].

The Effect of Postbiotics in the Improvement of Colorectal Cancer Therapies

Cancer is a public health concern and an emerging complication in developing countries, and also the second common disease that increases the mortality rates in the United States. It estimates that approximately 1,685,210 cases were expected recently, which is about 4,600 new cancer cases were diagnoses daily throughout the world. Colorectal cancer (CRC) is the third most common cancer diagnosed in women and men in the United States. Colorectal cancer in Malaysia, is considered the second most common cancer in men and women during 2016. Approximately 2000 cases in women and 2600 cases in men were reported in Malaysia with a 1000 and 1300 death rate, respectively [417]. Colorectal cancer mortality rates are elevating and have become the fourth leading cause of cancer fatalities throughout the world [418]. Nevertheless, the reported statistics of this cancer are underestimated in developed Asian countries such as South Korea, Japan, and Singapore in comparison to Malaysia and other developing countries. Diet has been demonstrated to decrease the incidence of CRC in a value of 80% due to its multiple impacts that could modify the host's metabolites composition or metabolome. Despite the advancement in cancer therapy and diagnosis, it has remained an important burden of disease all over the world which leads to the high incidence of mortality rated. Additionally, noxious side effects are generally pertinent to the chemotherapeutic agents currently available because of unspecific toxicity towards normal cells. Several health impacts are related to LAB and most of the researches on anticancer effects of LAB was extensively shown on colorectal cancer [419]. Fermented foods are rich in LAB abundantly, which are associated with vegetation, oral cavity, gastrointestinal (GI), and urogenital tract. These are commonly related to several health-promoting factors. The LAB's ability for serving as a food preservative is because of the production of the anti-microbial metabolite by targeting cell walls or membranes of the organisms like the bacteriocins and organic acids. Pyocin, colicin, and microcin as bacteriocins are considered inhibitory LAB-produced metabolites [420]. Their structure is consisting of amino acids that play an essential role in preventing the growth of the competing microorganism, and have been confirmed to have antineoplastic activity. Isolated L. plantarum I-UL4 from Malaysian fermented food, as Tapai Ubi that can produce compounds of bioactive metabolic as postbiotics [421]. UL4-PPM as a postbiotic or *L. plantarum* I-UL4-produced metabolite is believed to implement the probiotic impacts without living cells. Until now, not much investigation has been conducted about postbiotics and their metabolite products in cancer-related researches since it has been explained that LAB has anti-cancer properties by immune responses modulating *in-vivo* and *in vitro* investigations.

The Impact of Postbiotics on the Response to Visceral Pain Modulation

Irritable bowel syndrome (IBS) is a chronic disorder that has characterized by discomfort, abdominal pain, and visceral pain [422]. The magnitude of the autonomic response to visceral stimulation like the distension can be utilized in animal models for quantifying the visceral perception intensity and the visceral autonomic function [423]. It has been proposed that the administration of the probiotic can recuperate the IBS symptoms. An investigation conducted by Kamiya *et al.* (2006) demonstrated that probiotics or postbiotics derived from *L. reuteri* (heat or gamma-ray inactivated) in oral gavage form in rats (1×10^9 cells), 're able to inhibit the colorectal distension- visceral pain in rats.

The Effect of Postbiotics on the Respiratory System Functions

Postbiotics can be effective in treating and reducing the symptoms of respiratory diseases such as allergic inflammation of the nasal mucosa, colds, asthma, and pneumonia. Oral administration of postbiotic drops prepared from E*nterococcus faecalis* significantly reduced sneezing and itchy nose by modulating immune responses in guinea pigs with allergic inflammation of the nasal mucosa. The use of these postbiotics increases the regulatory T cells (CD25+, CD4+) in the spleen and reduces the entry of eosinophils into the mucosa, which ultimately suppresses IgE production and reduces the activity of eosinophils [394]. In a study on the elderly, it was found that the use of *Lactobacillus pentosus* derived postbiotics, along with optimal physical activity, increases the secretion of IgA in saliva [424]. It can also be effective in the elderly to improve the immune system's function against infections and reduces the incidence of colds [425].

The Effect of Postbiotics in the Reduction of the Aging Effects

In recent decades, aging-related diseases have increased for a variety of reasons. Memory impairment, decreased immune responses, increased peroxidation, and decreased bone density are considered complications of aging [133]. There are limited but satisfactory reports on the effect of postbiotics on the manifestations of aging [376, 426]. For example, it has been shown that the oral use of postbiotic meaningfully affects bone regeneration by influencing the population of osteoclasts in bone tissue [427]. Also, oral administration of postbiotics can boost cell-dependent immune systems in mice, which eventually alters the age-related aging process in the immune system [426]. Also, using postbiotics by improving the balance between Th1 and Th2 can prevent age-related diseases [133].

The Role of Postbiotics in the Reduction of Tooth Decay

Tooth decay is one of the most common chronic diseases in infancy. The disease begins with the initial dissolution of the tooth mineral and progresses to the local destruction of the enamel and dentin, which if left untreated, will lead to inflammation of the pulp and periapical. In this regard, *Streptococcus mutans* is known as the main microorganism found in most dental caries lesions. The strategy of using probiotics and postbiotics to improve oral health is a relatively new concept that has been studied extensively [428]. Research performed by Tanzer *et al*. on laboratory animals (mice) showed that adding the heat-inactivated *Lactobacillus paracasei* DSMZ16671 to a diet containing *Streptococcus mutans*, established a significant reduction in the dental caries rate of the investigated animals without adverse effects on the natural microbiota of the oral cavity. The results of this study showed that postbiotics can have a key role in the growth-stimulating of beneficial microbiota as well as an inhibitory role for pathogenic microorganisms. Therefore, they can prevent the complications and diseases caused by the growth and development of pathogenic germs in the oral cavity [429]. This provides an opportunity for the development of postbiotic products, which besides affecting the host's digestive system, can have therapeutic and health-promoting effects on other parts (oral cavity) of the body.

The Impact of Postbiotics on the Atopic Dermatitis Treatment

Atopic dermatitis (AD) is considered a chronic skin disorder with refractory properties that represent commonly itself itching eczema, including repeated regressions and exacerbations [430]. In the primary stage of AD, the skin barrier has broken and/or been injured because of eruption itching. It leads to an elevated rate in pro-inflammatory cytokines production that activates the immune system's various cells and triggering the inflammatory AD cycle [431]. AD is characterized through the denominated responses by T helper 2 cells. The immunoglobulin E production is mediated by Th2 cells as a result of cytokines releasing and other chemical mediators [432]. Some reports declare that probiotics can be utilized in AD treatment. One investigation demonstrates that probiotics and postbiotic derived from *L. sakei* prevent skin lesions and inflammation in rats. The treatment *via* probiotics and postbiotic of *L. sakei* probio-65 suspended in PBS (5×10^9 CFU/mL) decreases the lesions of skin and the itching frequency, the IgE levels, and the chemokines. Improving the skin lesions following treatment by probiotics and postbiotic derived from *L. sakei* probio-65 have an inhibitory impact on IgE and/or specific Th-2 cytokines (IL-4 & IL-6) [433]. Besides, Moroi *et al*. (2011) demonstrated that postbiotics from *L. paracasei* K71 [heat-inactivated, administered in powder form (2×10^{11} bacteria)] decrease the AD symptoms in elderly patients. Treatment *via* postbiotics decreases the severity of scores for the lesions of skin in comparison to the placebo group (non-treated group)[434]. Therefore, the biological responses in AD can be modified by postbiotics.

The Suppression Effect of Postbiotics and Age-Associated Manifestations

Age-related complications have more tendency to be aggravated because of the elderly population growth. Physiological phenomena related to aging include impairment of memory, a decrease in the immune response, *in vivo* peroxidation elevating, and bone density loss. Functional foods that contribute to aging control and extended health situations would be desirable. One investigation revealed that oral *Lac. lactis* subsp. *cremoris* H61 (heat-inactivated, lyophilized and added in the diet at 0.05% w/w) postbiotics administration to mice including accelerated senescence could overcome some age-related symptoms, like the hair loss, bone density loss, skin ulcers incidence, fecal *Staphylococcus* count and modifying the immune response through the production of higher IL-12 and IFN-γ. The postbiotics administration has the potency for preventing age-related disorders because of improving the balance between Th1 and Th2. It seems that the ability to overcome bone density loss is pertinent to the low osteoclast content. The osteoclast has a crucial role in the reabsorption of bone and therefore, this postbiotics consumption influence the reabsorption instead of bone formation [427].

Despite its current limitations, a metabolite-based therapeutic strategy is highly promising. In the next 5 years, microbiome researchers will need to include metabolomic characterization of the microbial ecosystem in their routine repertoire of tools, which will allow the community to define functional signatures for disease states that have so far been associated only with compositional and metagenomic changes. Simultaneously, the identification of new sensors for microbial metabolites will enable new insights into the mechanisms by which the activity of the microbial ecosystem is assessed by the host, with direct implications for the initiation of inflammation *versus* the maintenance of homeostasis. The discovery of novel sensors of metabolites will ultimately enable the targeted manipulation of the downstream signaling cascades in cases where the host has a disproportionate response to the microbiome.

CHAPTER 6

Perspectives on the Postbiotics Application

Abstract: Currently, bioactive compounds with health-promoting properties such as probiotics, prebiotics, and postbiotics have been gaining researchers' consideration. Probiotics and postbiotics are frequently employed in various pharmaceutical industries and/or commercial food-based crops. These bioactive elements can be related to the host eukaryotic cells and possess a vital role in keeping and reestablishing host health. Notwithstanding the efficiency of live probiotic cells, scientists have employed the novel concept of "postbiotic" to augment their advantageous effects as well as to meet the requirements of consumers to provide a safe product. The outcomes of recent investigations suggest that postbiotics might be a suitable substitute for live probiotics and can be used in medical, veterinary, and food practice to hinder and treat some diseases, enhance animal health status and develop functional foods. Currently, scientific reports approved that postbiotics, as a potential substitute, may possess superiority regarding safety issues compared to their parent probiotic cells, and because of their exclusive features in terms of technological, clinical, and economic aspects, can be employed as hopeful approaches in the drug and food industry for developing health benefits, and therapeutic targets. The chapter describes the potential applications of postbiotics in pharmaceutical formulations and commercial food-based crops for health advancement, hindrance of disease, and utilization as complementary treatments.

Keywords: Aquaculture, Complementary treatment, Disease resistance, Functional food, Immunomodulation, Pharmaceutical, Postbiotics, Probiotics, Prebiotics, Safety, Veterinary.

The growing information about functional foods has resulted in the development of novel products, such as those that contain probiotics. However, one concern associated with the probiotics application is the emerging antibiotic resistant genes in some probiotics strains. Probiotic cells can pass the antibiotic resistant genes to pathogenic microorganisms employing horizontal gene transfer [435]. Another critical issue linked to the product formulations of probiotics (*i.e.,* commercial food-based products and pharmaceutics) has maintained bacterial viability during the storage. The viability of probiotic cell in manufacturing products (*i.e.,* commercial food-based products or pharmaceutics), can be influenced *via* various variables such as communication with other present microbial species, products final acidity, temperature, water activity (aw),

Amin Abbasi, Elham Sheykhsaran & Hossein Samadi Kafil

nutrients obtainability, growth inhibitor, and promoter agents, level of inoculation, dissolved oxygen, fermentation period, and formulation method like the spray drying, freeze-drying, or freeze concentration [86, 436]. Moreover, differences between actual and stated probiotic quantities in joinery products for both veterinary and human usage have been explained previously [437]. Therefore, this lack of probiotic consistency presumably compromises the expected health profits generated by probiotic products.

In contrast, postbiotics are proposing to be higher consistent in comparison to the living bacteria as their sources. Phister, O'Sullivan, and McKay (2004) [438] showed that peptides with antimicrobial activity or chloromethane and bacilysin, derived from *Bacillus* sp. strain CS93 are water-soluble and active higher than a broad pH range, which can extend their application in a broad variety of food products. Moreover, utilizing selected lactic acid bacteria that produce phytase as starters to bread-making have been displayed as appropriate alternatives to prepare whole wheat bread, including low phytate content [439]. Nevertheless, earlier investigations have demonstrated that phytate advanced hydrolysis has acquired by elevating the fermentation time and/or reducing the pH in the fermentation of whole wheat dough; situations that not only probably act as an influencing g factor in sensory attributes of the final products, but can affect the phytate degrading enzymes synthesis by microorganisms [440]. With the utilizing purified enzymes degrading by phytate, these components would not be considered a critical challenge. Another important beneficial effect of postbiotics is safety profile as no requirement to uptake countless living microbes [441]. Moreover, postbiotics can be utilized in a standardized and controlled condition, whereas, in the living bacteria application cases, the active structure level in the gut is depending on the metabolic activity and the number of respective strains [442]. Therefore, a great concern is scientific knowledge translation into commercial applications and create a bridge between industry and science (Table 7).

PHARMACEUTICAL APPLICATIONS

At present, cell-free preparations acquired from the metabolic products belong to various useful bacteria have been shown with broad applications in the pharmaceutical scope as a preventative agent or treatment of complications [444]. For example, Colibiogen® (Laves-Arzneimittel GmbH, Schötz, Switzerland) as a well-known commercially protein-free filtrate based on the *Escherichia coli* (strain Laves 1931) cultures, contains peptides, amino acids, fatty acids, and polysaccharides which are effective in the *in vitro* inhibition both antibiotic-resistant and sensitive *Salmonella* isolates [445], in the murine colitis recuperation [446], and to remarkably decreasing skin lesions in polymorphous light eruptions-patients [447]. A bacteria-free liquid containing metabolic products is Hylak® Forte (Ratiopharm/Merckle GmbH, Germany) (*e.g.* SCFA, lactic acid other non-identified metabolites) derived from *Streptococcus faecalis* DSM 4086, *L. helveticus* DS 4183, *E. coli* DSM 4087, and *L. acidophilus* DSM 414 has been approved to be useful in the salmonellosis management in infants [448] and the intestinal dysbacteriosis of patients with chronic gastritis treatment [449]. Additionally, it has been demonstrated to remarkably decreasing the severity and incidence of radiation-induced diarrhea in radio-oncology-patients [450]. CytoFlora® (BioRay Inc., Laguna Hills, CA, USA), as a micronized cell wall lysates preparation of *B. longum, B. infantis, B. bifidum, L. sporogenes,L. acidophilus* DDS-1*, L. casei, L. salivarius, L. bulgaricus, L. reuteri, L. plantarum, S. thermophilus, L. acidophilus,* and *L. rhamnosus* that has been utilizing for correcting gut dysbiosis, a well-adjusted immune response improvement, and recuperating autistic children's symptoms [451]. Del-Immune V® (Pure Research Products, LLC, Boulder, CO, USA), is considered as another commercial product as a US Food and Drug Administration-registered formulation containing amino acids, muramyl peptides, and DNA fragments derived from *L. rhamnosus* V (DV strain), has demonstrated to remarkably decreasing the gastrointestinal distress severity in Autism Spectrum Disorder- children if administrated as a blend of Del-Immune V® plus probiotics [452] (Fig. 7).

Table 7. Some of the best-known postbiotics [443].

Name	Contents and Properties
Hylak forte (Germany)	Liquid pharmaceutical comprising no microbial cells and administrated orally. It includes postbiotic products generated by the following strains: *Streptococcus faecalis* DSM 4086 (12.5g/100ml), *Lactobacillus acidophilus* DSM 4149 (12.5g/100ml), *Lactobacillus helveticus* DSM 4183 (50g/100ml) and *Escherichia coli* DSM 4087 (25g/100ml). The health-promoting properties of this postbiotic in kids and adults is related to the amendment of gut microbiota functions and composition, normalization of vitamin B and K levels in a microorganism, supplying enterocytes and immune intestinal cells with energy, acid-alkaline balance, and water-salt balance. The positive properties of this sterile pharmaceutical liquid are explained *via* the attendance of a complex of lactic acid, volatile fatty acids, and some undefined low molecular microbial constituents.
Bactistatin (Russia)	The powdered cultural liquid of *Bacillus subtilis*, comprising inactivated bacteria and a collection of several low molecular weight constituents, metabolites and natural sorbent zeolite.
Colibiogen (Switzerland)	The filtered cultural liquid of *Escherichia coli* (strain *Laves* 1931), comprising peptides, amino acids, polysaccharides, and fatty acids.
Pro-Symbioflor (Germany)	Germ-free lysate and cultural fluid of *E.coli* and *Enterococcus faecalis*.

(Table 7) cont.....

Name	Contents and Properties
Helinorm (Germany/Russia)	Deactivated probiotic cells (*L.reuteri)* that connection precisely to *H. pylori* and remove these bacteria obviously from the organism; suggested for gastric ulcer, cancer prevention and gastritis.
CytoFlora (USA)	The lysates of cell-wall of *B. infantis, B. longum, B. bifidum, L. salivarius, L. reuteri, L. bulgaris, L. casei,* and *Streptococcus thermophiles.*
Del-Immune V (USA)	DNA fragments and peptidoglycans of *L. rhamnosus.*
Daigo (Japan)	A combination of biocontroller protein fractions derived from cultural fluids of various *lactobacilli L.curvatus, L.fermentum, L.acidophilus, L.rhamnosus, L.casei, L.plantarum, L.brevis,* and *L.salivarius* after a yearly cultivating on soymilk.
Complex functional foods fortifier (Russia)	The filtered *Bifidobacterium longum* B 379 M and *Lactobacillus acidophilus* NK-1 cultured on particular milk medium and removal of live cells were achieved through microfiltration; contains organic acids, micro- and macro-molecules, amino acids, and B vitamins. It is a multifaceted strengthener, and the products resulting from its use are described by metabolic activity and a significant effect on the host. Applied as a main or ancillary constituent (in the native or powder form, or as a concentrate) in the creation of numerous types of beverages.
"New Class of Pharmabiotic" (Russia)	Generated by *Streptococcus thermophilus,* and lactobacilli (three strains) in a long fermentation from raw materials such as fruit, herbs, berries, vegetables, and animal products. A mechanical process (centrifugation) applied to elimination of unfermented peptides, amino acids, sediments, volatile organic acids, vitamins, proteases, and microelements composed in the liquid portion. The produced product has numerous beneficial effects on host health.

It has been shown that cell lysates of probiotics presumably are containing sphingomyelinase, hyaluronic acid, exopolysaccharides, lipoteichoic acid, peptidoglycan, acetic acid, lactic acid, and/or diacetyl, with a wide ability to provide a biologic activity that can harness to obtain skin advantages like the improvement of atopic dermatitis, atopic eczema, burns and scars healing, properties of skin-rejuvenating, skin innate immunity improving and protecting against photodamage [453]. Based on it, several investigations and patents have been reporting on utilizing extracts of probiotics for developing personal care products such as skin products, oral, and underarm (deodorants and antiperspirants) [454 - 456]. Functions of mitochondria, oxidative stress, and lipid metabolism were investigating, employing spectrophotometric, Seahorse analyzer, and biochemical determinations. Besides, liver protection through the NaB has been investigated in VPA-treated epileptic WAG/Rij-rats, after receiving NaB for six months.

The data displayed that NaB prevents VPA toxicity, cell oxidative limitation, and mitochondrial destruction (malondialdehyde, ROS, SOD activity, and bioenergetics of mitochondria), and restoration of fatty acid oxidation in HepG2 cells (the activity of carnitine palmitoyl-transferase and peroxisome proliferator-activated receptor α expression), isolated mitochondria, and primary hepatocytes. These results enforce the protective abilities of NaB on VPA-induced liver damage and demonstrating it as an appropriate therapeutic strategy in counteracting general side effects because of VPA chronic treatment.

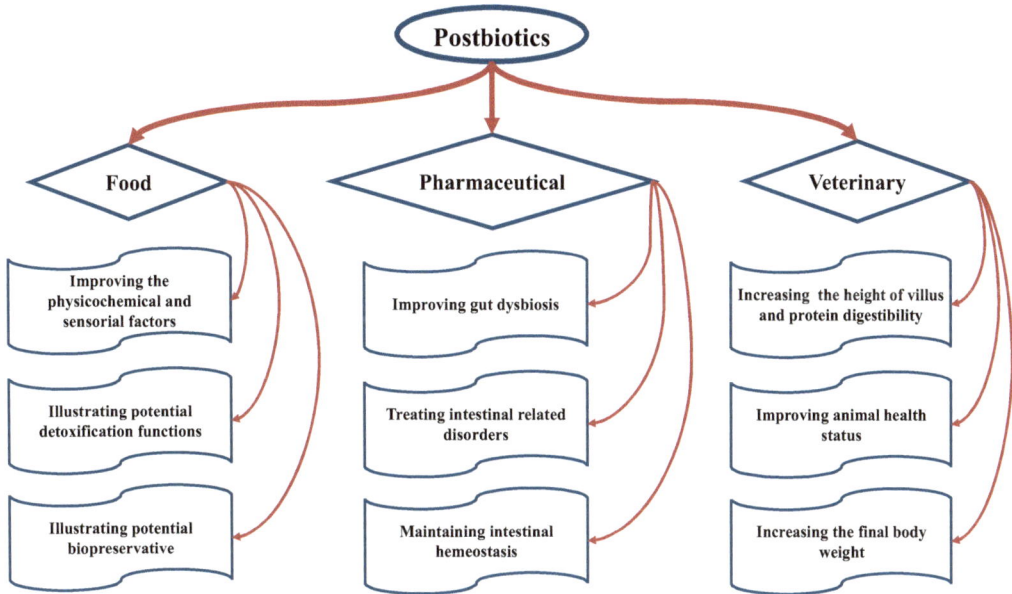

Fig. (7). The main application of postbiotics in pharmaceutical, veterinary and food practices.

Alopecia areata (AA) or 'area Celsi', is considered the second common form of hair loss that affects the scalp. Recently suggested treatments for AA therapy include low-level light form, biologics like the inhibitors of Janus kinase, and autologous platelet-rich plasma (PRP), as a well-known "elixir" for hair growth . Developing bioactive peptides has been conducted employing applications of biotechnology materials it acts for overcoming the PRP limitations. In recent years, the microbiota involvement in hair growth complications, particularly in AA has been shown, and the advantages of microbial metabolites (postbiotics) have been demonstrated as well. Rinaldi *et al.*, (2020) as designers of a randomized double-blinded parallel-group research in which 160 individuals (male and female) were influenced by AA and their age range was 18 to 60 years. In this investigation, the randomized subjects were allocated to a treatment group (group 1), TR-PRP plus-Celsi received the cosmetic product, and a placebo group (group 2). The Severity of Alopecia Tool or SALT score was obtained in two groups at baseline and following 2- 3 months of treatment, and the data in comparison to two groups. The data approved the positive effect of postbiotics, hence the group 1 subjects demonstrated a remarkable modification from baseline in SALT score in 2 months during the treatment (61.04% ± 3.45%; p\0.0001), with more improvement at the final treatment (3 months) (69.56% ± 4.32%; p\0.0001). No remarkable modifications from baseline were observed for the group 2 subjects (T1: 26.45% ± 3.64%; T3: 27.63% ± 7.61%). The data in this research provide more proof of the efficacy of the bioactive peptides which mimic the growth factors currently exist in PRP in AA-influenced subjects. They were added to our existing knowledge of the association between hair growth complications and microbiota, and emphasize the significant role of investigations about the microbial community and microbial metabolites as an emerging therapeutic approach [458].

The neuropeptide hormone oxytocin plays a critical role in energy metabolism, social bonding, and wound healing as an appropriate physical point, and social and mental health. It was demonstrated previously that *Lactobacillus reuteri* is a proper source of commensal microbe for human feeding and adequate for endogenous oxytocin levels up-regulation and improving factor in wound healing ability in mice. Varian *et al*., (2016), report that oral *L. reuteri* can induce skin wound repairing and extend to human cases as well. Moreover, supplementation of diet including a sterile lysate of microbe is adequate for levels of oxytocin, boosts systemic, and promotes wound repairing ability. Oxytocin-producing cells in mouse models were observing to be elevated in the caudal paraventricular nucleus [PVN] of the hypothalamus following the feeding of the preparation of a sterile lysed *L. reuteri*, coincident with stress hormone's blood levels in few amounts of corticosterone and higher rapid epidermal closures. The researchers conclude that the viability of microbes is not crucial to regulate the host's oxytocin levels and the bacterial postbiotics presumably modulate oxytocin secretion of the host for personalized health subjects and the potential public [459].

Intestinal commensal bacteria can generate bioactive molecules with entrance ability into circulation and influence of host homeostasis and physiology. However, there is little knowledge about the ability of these metabolites for crossing the blood-brain barrier (BBB) and entrance into the developing brain under a common physiological situation. Swann *et al*., (2020), applied a liquid chromatography-mass spectrometry-based metabolomics access for characterizing the microbial-derived metabolites' developmental profiles in the mice's forebrains across three key postnatal developmental steps, co-occurrence with the gut microbiota maturation. They showed that direct metabolites of the intestinal microbiome such as imidazole propionate or the combinatorial metabolism products between the host and microbiome such as trimethylamine-N-oxide, 3-indoxyl-sulfate and, phenyl acetyl glycine) currently exist in the mice's forebrains as primary as the neonatal period and remains until elderly ages. The researchers proposed that the biomolecules derived from microbes can cross the BBB both in detection form and as precursor molecules undergoing more processing in the brain. These chemical messengers can attach to the receptors which are expressed in the brain. Hence, modifications in the gut microbiome presumably affect the neurodevelopmental trajectories through microbial-associated metabolites regulation [460].

APPLICATION IN VETERINARY SCOPE

Improving animal health is considered a promising point of utilizing due to the reports of postbiotics probable influencing role in the growth performance of broilers, hens, and piglets [461, 462]. In this regard, a recent investigation conducted by Kareem *et al.* (2016a) revealed that postbiotics- fed (generated from *L. plantarum*)broilers developed remarkably more final body weight and total weight gain in comparison to the basal diet- fed broilers without postbiotics. Also, postbiotics have remarkable increasing ileal and duodenal villus height [461]. Furthermore, the postbiotics in part with inulin probably promote growth performance, the final count of useful bacteria, and decrease the *E. coli* and *Enterobacteria* population's presence [463]. In a similar investigation, Loh *et al.* (2014) showed a remarkable hen's daily higher production of hen's egg per day if a postbiotic supplement was administrated. Some literature suggested that the administration of *L. plantarum* postbiotics implement a positive impact on protein digestibility and growth performance, as well as decreased incidence of diarrhea. According to the collected information, the authors proposed that postbiotics change the architecture of mucus in terms of promoted animal growth performance and longer villi. Besides, utilizing postbiotics modify the gut microbiota, promotes the protective bacteria (*e.g.*, *Lactobacillus* and *Bifidobacterium*) population, and improves the health conditions of the subject animals. Additionally, postbiotics have contained antimicrobial compounds generated by *Lactobacillus* strains, which probably provide nutrients and improve the physiological activities in the animal's gut, these interactions lead to the improvement of absorption and reducing gut pathogenic bacteria. Postbiotics can be regarded as potential contributors and feed additives for achieving appropriate animal health and more productivity [464].

The Potential Application of Postbiotics in Aquaculture

The application of probiotics is well-established in the aquaculture area. However, this procedure is yet to take the momentum. After the primary investigation by Villamil *et al.* (2002), it was revealed that the immune-stimulatory benefits of *Lactococcus lactis* were killed by heat in turbot, plenty of preparations of postbiotic have been examined on shellfish and fish. These researches were conducted to survey the impacts of postbiotics in immune responses mediating, growth, and disorder resistance [465]. Several investigations have revealed that the postbiotics have equal benefits like their viable forms in immunity modulating and providing disorder resistance [267, 466]. In contrast, viable useful microbes can provide better health-promoting effects in comparison to their non-viable counterparts [272].

Immunostimulation

The postbiotics stimulation role in the immune system has been studied completely in the higher vertebrate model [133]. Investigations have been conducted on shellfish and fish and their immunity stimulation potency both under *in vivo* and *in vitro* conditions is remarkable. The postbiotic ability in immune response stimulation has been examined employing the *in vitro* model by many researchers. For instance, the remarkable activity of enhanced respiratory burst, phagocytic activity, production of nitric oxide, and the proliferative response has been shown in fish head-kidney leukocytes exposed to different *in vitro* postbiotic preparations [268, 269]. *In vitro* up-regulated expression of several immune-related genes such as pro-inflammatory cytokines [IL-1 (IL-1b), IL-17A/F-3, IL-8, IL-6, TNF- (TNF-N and TNF-a) and COX-2], antibacterial epinecidin-1, cell-mediated immune regulators [IL-12p40, IL-12p35, and IL-18], antiviral cytokines [IFNc and I-IFN], other regulatory cytokines [IL-7, IL-2, IL-21, IL-15, IL-10, and TGF-b1], TLR2 and IgM have been reported as well [273, 467]. Besides, other defense genes expression viz. bactericidal permeability-increasing protein/lipopolysaccharide-binding protein (BPI/LBP), catalase, g-type lysozyme, non-specific cytotoxic cell receptor protein-1, phospholipid-hydroperoxide glutathione peroxidase, and granzyme A/K were remarkably up-regulated after postbiotics *in vitro* exposure to fish head-kidney leukocytes [468].

Postbiotics *in vivo* administration has been shown to stimulate several humoral and cellular immune responses such as the activity of gut lysozyme and serum, production of oxygen radicals, the activity of peroxidase myeloperoxidase, natural hemolytic complement, and alkaline phosphatase, a1-antiprotease, and levels of immunoglobulin and total serum protein in different fish species [469, 470]. Also, a remarkable raising in the macrophages number, populations of lymphocyte, acidophilic granulocytes, and IgM+ cells in the gut, neutrophils migration, bactericidal activity of plasma, phagocytic activity, respiratory burst, and cytotoxic activity have been shown in exposed fish to daily dietary postbiotics [277, 466]. As regards the immune-relevant genes expression, the postbiotic diet can instigate the pro-inflammatory cytokines (IL-6, IL-1b, IL-17A/F-3, TNF-a, and TNF-N) expression, cell-mediated immune regulators (IL-12p40, IL-12p35, and IL-18), antiviral cytokines (IFNc and I-IFN-1), and other regulatory cytokines (IL-2, IL-7, IL-21, IL-10, and TGF-b1), TLR2, C3 and genes of iNOS [267, 470]. Remarkable promotion in immune parameters viz. total hemocyte count, respiratory burst activity, and phenoloxidase was shown in giant freshwater prawn (*Macrobrachium rosenbergii*) fed with *L. plantarum* killed by heat [267]. Another research has reported that, dead (heat-killed and sonicated) *L. plantarum* increases the prophenoloxidase, superoxide dismutase, and lysozyme gene expression of white leg shrimp (*Litopenaeus vannamei*) under the condition of acute low salinity stress [270]. All published reports show a potential useful impact of postbiotics in immunostimulation at the molecular and cellular level. The peroxidase myeloperoxidase immunostimulatory properties presumably are due to bacterial cell's different structural components. Previous studies have shown the bacterial cell's several chemical compounds involve in the immune responses [381]. However, more researches must be conducting to delineating the action's precise mechanism.

Growth

The digestive tract's metabolic functions in aquatic animals maybe are affected by indigenous microbiota positively [471]. Furthermore, there are pieces of evidence that live useful microbes (feed probiotics) elevate the aquatic animals' appetite through the digestibility improving [469]. Similar to probiotics, postbiotics can promote the growth performance and feed application of aquatic animals. For instance, postbiotic (*L. plantarum*) killed by heat has been shown to remarkably elevate the feed application and growth performance of red seabream (*Pagrus major*) [472]. Rodriguez-Estrada *et al.* (2013) showed the remarkable elevating in specific growth rate (SGR), weight gain (WG), feed increment, and efficiency of protein ratio (PER) of rainbow trout (*Oncorhynchus mykis*) fed with cells of *Enterococcus faecalis* inactivated by heat [473]. Dietary *Bacillus pumilus* probiotic inactivated by heat remarkably promoted the WG, final weight, and SGR of grouper (*Epinephelus coioides*) juveniles [274]. In a recent investigation, Zheng *et al.* (2017) reported the increasing rate in white leg shrimp's growth parameters when fed with sonicated *L. plantarum* killed by heat [270]. In contrast, *B. subtilis, L. lactis, and S. cerevisiae* heat-killed probiotics in rohu's diet did not impart any remarkable growth changes, nutrient retention, PER, digestibility, the ratio of feed conversion, and colonization of the gut [474]. Similarly, *L. plantarum* heat-killed feed supplements did not change the giant freshwater prawn's growth parameters [267]. Postbiotics can affect positively different fish's growth parameters but the mechanism of action is still not well-understood.

Disease Resistance

Postbiotics influence the host beneficially through the recuperating resistance of disease against the infections caused by pathogens. Although the postbiotics pathogen-inhibiting mechanisms are not well-understood, presumably the immunostimulation is a principal mode of conferring resistance-action to the host against pathogenic microorganisms. An *in vitro* investigation by Villamil *et al.* (2002) reported remarkable *Vibrio anguillarum* growth inhibition as a pathogen incubated with heat-killed lactic acid bacteria [465]. *A. salmonicida*-infected rainbow trout mortality rates were remarkably decreased in the case of formalin-killed postbiotic feeding [473]. The formalin-killed commercial probiotic feeding to Nile tilapia (*Oreochromis niloticus*) leads to promoted resistance to infection caused by *Edwardsiella tarda* [475]. *Bacillus subtilis* AB1 (formalin-killed and sonicated) as a postbiotic can remarkably elevate the rainbow trout survivability, which is challenged with *Aeromonas* spp. as pathogens experimentally [476]. *Clostridium butyricum* killed by heat increases the Chinese Drum (*Miichthys miiuy*) survivability against infections caused by *A. hydrophila* and *V. anguillarum* [277]. In another research, pathogenic resistance to *V. harveyi* had been reported in Japanese pufferfish (*Takifugu rubripes*), which is treated with *L. plantarum* and heat-killed *L. paracasei* spp. *paracasei* [276]. Postbiotic obtained from *Enterobacter* spp. (Formalin-killed) decreases mortality rates of infections caused by *Flavobacterium psychrophilum* in rainbow trout [477]. Additionally, dietary heat-killed *L. plantarum* remarkably decreases the cumulative mortality rates of infections caused by *M. rosenbergii* and *A. hydrophila* [267]. The major part of these investigations reported immune responses' concurrent enhancement, implying the possible involvement of postbiotics' immunostimulatory properties for enhancing disease resistance.

FOOD APPLICATIONS

Even though many foods are ample naturally in postbiotics (*e.g.*, kefir, kombucha, yogurt, and pickled vegetables) or their precursors [478], some postbiotics utilize intentionally in special foods considering their production *in situ* through the producer strain. For example, cell-free supernatant derived from *L. Plantarum* YML007 has been considering soybeans grains bio-preservativ [479]. EPS contains infrequent sugars is an interesting topic for new utilization in the food industry because of their physicochemical role (stabilizing, viscosifying, or water-binding capacities), and sensorial (palatability) properties in the final food products; nevertheless, except for dextran, EPS derived from lactic acid bacteria have not been still commercially actuated as food additives due to their low yields [480]. Nisin as a specific *Lactococcus lactis* suspend *Lactis* lantibiotic is the only bacteriocin that has been confirmed to be utilized as a food preservative. Examples of food products with Nisin are included ice for storing fresh fish, baby foods, canned soups, baked goods, mayonnaise, and dairy products, particularly cheeses [481]. Regarding the above mentions, the utilizing of foods as a postbiotics delivery system appears to contains a field with many opportunities, however with major concerns.

Although the beneficial effects of health have been associating with postbiotics, most information in the literature demonstrates these beneficial impacts are related to their direct consumption. Hence, the application of the food as delivery vehicles for postbiotics seems to constitute an explored field for many opportunities and issues, including I) probiotic species and strains selection for production of postbiotic, II) implement of adequate techniques for delivery and inactivation, III) investigation of their activity and consistency in food shelf life, and IV) use of proper methodologies to investigate their biological impacts. For a broad postbiotics application, the first concern is the deal with the proper probiotic species and strains selection that are considering current specific health beneficial effects, which are retaining to an acceptable level of obtained postbiotics. Secondly, many inactivated conditions have been applied for obtaining postbiotics, it is not well-understood that all cases are proper for all species/strains and food applications or not. A serious concern is the impact determination of the inactivation method on the consistency of the postbiotics beneficial effects throughout their shelf life. It is utmost of importance to define the postbiotics form(s) and their commercialization and ability for delivering health advantage if consumed with foods in all their shelf life. For example, postbiotics can be obtained as powders or liquid. In the case of the powder, which is the best candidate as a carrier? Have they potency to be commercialized at room temperature or must they be frozen? All mentioned aspects in the host must be investigated taking into consideration the health benefits retention. If postbiotics had the potency to be commercialized as consistent powders at room temperature, it would consider as an important benefit for their broad application in foods. A final requirement is to define the measuring mechanism of postbiotics biological activity to estimate their shelf lives and providing ways for assessing how a portion of food carries health advantages provided by postbiotics. If the delivering ability of health advantages in the hosts could be measured through methods such as flow cytometry or others, it would constitute an important advancement in terms of the postbiotics practical application in foods. These techniques have also gained major importance for postbiotics quality control. Furthermore, to widespread using of postbiotics in foods, a few situations must be investigated like the ease of production (easy method for inactivation, that is cheap, controlled, and quick), proper solubility in foods, no or decreased interaction with foods, and consistency during the process and foods storage. Last but not least, the mechanism elucidation of postbiotics action, including the specific active components determination accounts for the useful impacts, comprising fundamental knowledge for allowing not only the postbiotics application in foods but also their health authorities' regulation [133, 134]. Additionally, the advent of modern genetic manipulation methods has provided opportunities for developing emerging bioengineered probiotic strains' capacity to generate preventative metabolites targeted to the treatment of several complications [482]. For example, genetically modified lactic acid bacteria are utilized to deliver intestinal antimicrobial peptides [483], angiotensin-converting enzyme inhibitory peptides [484], cancer-suppressing peptide KiSS1 [485], the HSP65 as a fusion protein with tandem repeats of P277 [486], and IL-10 cytokine and glutamic acid decarboxylase [487], therefore, promising strategies provision for hypertension, enteric infections, colon carcinoma, and intestinal inflammatory and autoimmune diseases treatment like the Type 1 diabetes mellitus. Despite the beneficial biomedical application of recombinant probiotic metabolites, remarkable safety and aspects of the regulation still require to be investigated in depth.

As mentioned earlier in chapter one, various factors including increased prevalence of infectious and non-infectious diseases, high treatment costs, adverse effects of anticancer therapeutics, and so on result in modifications in people's lifestyles. Besides, to overcome the unfavorable effects of live probiotics, there is a growing desire for safe pharmaceutical or food products. In this regard, postbiotics gained much attention and are considered novel microbial-based approaches in the pharmaceutical and/or food industry. Further *in vitro*/*in vivo* experiments and clinical trials are required to define novel postbiotics and examine their safety parameters and stability in various health and disease conditions.

CHAPTER 7

The Challenges and Strategies to Add Postbiotic Components into Food Matrices

Abstract: The matrix of foods and beverages (fermented or/and non-fermented), especially those considered a regular part of the daily diet, are genuine options to add postbiotic ingredients for carrying them. Along with increasing consumer knowledge about the health-promoting effects of functional foods, their demands rise. Hence, in the industrial sector, its promotion is also appreciated. Over the past two decades, as researchers have focused on bioactive compounds, many of these compounds have been identified. Still, despite extensive research, a small number of these compounds have been successfully incorporated into the functional food matrix. It indicates the need for more knowledge and investigation to study the nature of the bioactive compound and high-performance biotechnology methods to using these compounds in the food industry. In this case, postbiotic compounds were also in the early stages of their entry into the food industry, and for a successful presence in this field, they face technological, legal, and commercial challenges. Consequently, understanding the characteristics of postbiotic compounds and nanostructure carriers is essential for designing the best delivery system. This chapter provides an overview of the challenges and strategies for adding postbiotic compounds into the food matrix.

Keywords: Biotechnology, Bioavailability, Delivery system, Food industry, Functional foods, Nanoencapsulation, Postbiotics.

The matrix of foods and beverages (fermented or/and non-fermented), especially those considering a regular part of the daily diet, are genuine options to add postbiotic ingredients for carrying them. Along with increasing consumer knowledge about the health-promoting effects of functional foods, their demands rise. Hence, in the industrial sector, its promotion is also appreciated [488]. Considering the needs of society and consumers is one of the fundamental factors in developing functional food products. Scientific reports indicate a lack of nutrients or an increase in the prevalence of a particular disease in a geographical area. However, researchers are working to develop beneficial products with a focus on bioactive compounds that play a significant role in compensating for nutrient deficiencies or treating diseases [18].

Amin Abbasi, Elham Sheykhsaran & Hossein Samadi Kafil

Some parameters such as a) production efficiency, b) storage stability, c) easy distribution, d) and raised demands from the community to provide a safe product, are substantial factors for producers in this industry [489]. The appropriate performance of functional food (*e.g.*, a food matrix containing postbiotic components) that links to specified clinical conditions can raise its acceptance as a dietary supplement by consumers. Over the past two decades, as researchers have focused on bioactive compounds, many of these compounds have been identified. But despite extensive research, a small number of these compounds have been successfully incorporated into the functional food matrix. It indicates the need for more knowledge and investigation to study the nature of the bioactive compound and high-performance biotechnology methods to using these compounds in the food industry. In this case, postbiotic compounds were also in the early stages of their entry into the food industry. For a successful presence in this field, they face technological, legal, and commercial challenges.

APPROPRIATE FOOD CARRIER FOR POSTBIOTIC COMPOUNDS

Some factors, such as the structure and shape of the food carrier for postbiotic compounds are very important in the process of producing functional foods. For the development of postbiotic products, fundamental factors such as physical, chemical, and biological properties of postbiotic components, also their effect on taste, texture and stability, processing conditions, and acceptance of the final product should all be considered in developing the formulation of these products. Also, other main factors such as the solubility properties of postbiotics, their stability, and sensorial factors should be considered in the selection of appropriate food carriers, in which case, the postbiotic components can be added to solid, semi-solid, powdered, or liquid foods [490, 491].

THE ISSUES RELATED TO THE ADDITION OF BIOACTIVE COMPOUNDS (POSTBIOTICS) INTO THE FOOD MATRIX

The process of enrichment or the addition of bioactive components into the food matrix is intricate. The enrichment of a new element to a product can cause a dramatic effect on its structure, physicochemical, and shelf-life properties. On the other hand, the type and solubility of postbiotics significantly affect the design of the formulation and processing used in its production. In most cases, it is not possible to incorporate these compounds directly into the food matrix because they are sensitive to decomposition and may interact with other food ingredients, resulting in loss of bioavailability of the added component and reduced quality of the food product [492].

Therefore, the successful incorporation of postbiotic components into the food matrix requires the appropriate design of a carrier system that is specifically designed for the target product and maintains the functionality of added bioactive components (postbiotics).

CURRENT CHALLENGES

The need for a specific and impressive amount of postbiotic to have a known beneficial clinical effect is a fundamental challenge. Other challenges include preventing adverse interactions of postbiotics with other food matrix compounds, limiting the breakdown of the additive component (postbiotic) under food processing conditions, stabilizing the additive component during the storage, and ensuring that the final product contains a sufficient amount of postbiotic components and provides the desired health effect after digestion [493].

Bioactive compounds are unstable when extracted from their natural resources and cannot be added directly into the food matrix. Also, there is a wide range of biological elements among the postbiotic components with different physicochemical properties that can't easily add to the food matrix. On the other hand, various biotechnological methods with high compatibility and efficiency can use to successfully incorporate these components into the food matrix without any side-effect on the physicochemical, rheological, and sensorial aspects of the product [491]. The selection of appropriate food carriers, method, and time to add the additive component to stabilize during production, storage, distribution, and gastrointestinal conditions are among the important and effective factors in the bioavailability of postbiotic components.

THE BIOAVAILABILITY OF POSTBIOTICS

The bioavailability of a bioactive compound (postbiotic) depends on the changes that occur during its storage process in the food matrix and the passage of the gastrointestinal tract. The biological functions of bioactive compounds are significantly influencing by their pharmacokinetics (*e.g.* adsorption, distribution, metabolism, and excretion) [494]. The chemical structure of a compound affects the intensity and rate of absorption and the nature of plasma derivatives or metabolites. The adsorption rate affects bioavailability, so it determines how much bioactive compound (postbiotic) is available at the site of action and distributes to the organs after uptake.

It is noteworthy that the chemical structure, their interaction with food constituents, and gut microbiota are significantly affected their functionality. The delivery evaluation of various systems for the efficiency improvement of postbiotic components is often basing on the *in-vitro* , cell culture, and *in-vivo* models [495]. On the other hand, the host endogenous physiological environments' complexity (*in-vivo*) relative to the external environment (*in-vitro*) requires further communication and optimization between these two environments. Researchers should also consider this issue when considering the relationship between different external models and endogenous conditions. Delivery systems can provide an impressive tool for improving the efficiency and bioavailability of postbiotic compounds, but so far, no public delivery system has been introducing to carry all bioactive compounds.

THE STRATEGY OF THE ADDITION OF BIOACTIVE COMPOUNDS (POSTBIOTICS) INTO THE FOOD MATRIX

The encapsulation process is one of the most common methods for trapping bioactive agents in the matrix of carrier agent and also this method is considered a powerful tool to optimizing the delivery process of bioactive substances (*e.g.* antioxidants, minerals, vitamins, phytosterols, lutein, fatty acids, and lycopene) and living cells such as probiotics in the food matrix [496]. The encapsulation process can be defined as the technique of coating materials inside small capsules, as the digestive process continues, these capsules release their contents (postbiotics) in certain amounts over time in the target areas.

The encapsulation technique acts *via* separating the reactive components of postbiotics from other food systems' elements and controls their release [497]. The material used in the capsules' shell design must be edible, biodegradable, and create an impermeable membrane between the capsules' inner phase and its surrounding. In this regard, various compounds such as polysaccharides, proteins, and lipids are applied, as the most materials, in the encapsulation. Which usually maintains the natural properties of the product over time. Table **8** illustrates the most materials used for the encapsulation of bioactive components in the food industry.

Table 8. Most materials used for the encapsulation of bioactive components in the food industry.

Compounds	Types
Proteins	Milk proteins (whey protein isolates, caseinates, micellar casein, serum albumin, beta-lactoglobulin, lactoferrin, and alpha-lactalbumin), plant proteins (soy protein isolate, wheat protein, oatmeal protein, corn protein), and gelatine.
Carbohydrates	Sugars (glucose, sucrose, lactose, trehalose, glucose syrup, honey, oligosaccharides), starch and starch derivatives (natural, modified starch, resistant starch, maltodextrin), non starch polysaccharides (alginate, pectin, carrageenan, chitosan, plant fibers, gum arabic, xanthan, cellulose materials), cyclodextrins (beta-cyclodextrin and gamma-cyclodextrin).
Fats and waxes	Milk fat and milk fat fractions (olein and stearin), vegetable fats and oils (soybean oil, canola, palm oil, sunflower, and its fractions), waxes (such as carnauba, candelilla, and beeswax)

(Table 8) cont.....

Compounds	Types
Surface-active agents	Synthetic (tweens, spans, polyglycerol, sucrose esters), natural (milk phospholipids, soy phospholipids, saponins), mono- and di-glycerides (glycerol monostearate).

Micro/Nanoencapsulation techniques were developed to incorporate bioactive compounds to prevent adverse chemical reactions and their controlled release. In this regard, nanocarrier systems can divide into three groups based on wall material; nanocarriers based on lipids and surfactants, nanocarriers based on polysaccharides, and nanocarriers based on proteins. Lipid and surfactant-based nanocarriers include nanoliposomes, nanoemulsions, solid lipid nanoparticles (SLN), nanostructured lipid carriers (NLC), and micelles. Polysaccharide-based nanocarriers include polysaccharide nanoparticles and micelles. Protein-based nanocarriers also include casein micelles and various complex proteins such as albumin, gelatin, milk serum protein, whey protein, soy protein, and corn [494]. The use of nanocarriers for hydrophobic postbiotic compounds such as fat-soluble vitamins can have several benefits such as controlling its release at a given location and time, the stability of these compounds against light, heat, and oxygen during storage, increasing the solubility of hydrophobic compounds in the aquatic environment such as dairy products and beverages, increasing bioavailability and reducing the lack of product transparency due to their small size [498]. Although the nanoencapsulation technique increases the permeability of water-insoluble compounds, it shouldn't adversely affect the color, taste, and sensory properties of the product. The maintenance of the encapsulated bioactive compounds (postbiotic) during the production process as well as storage conditions should be done at the highest possible level, and in return, its release rate in the desired absorption location should be done optimally. It should be noted that the used delivery system should be compatible with other ingredients in the food matrix and should not adversely affect the physicochemical, qualitative properties (appearance, texture, and taste) as well as the acceptance of the final functional food product [499]. Since each of these systems has different benefits, such as the efficiency of capsulation, particle stability, aqueous solubility, oral absorption, and bioavailability, thus it is essential to understand the characteristics of postbiotic compounds and nanocarrier systems to design the best delivery system for each postbiotic components (Fig. **8**).

The Need to Issue a Permit for the Entry of Functional Postbiotic Foods into the Market and Monitor of them

According to the definition, functional foods commonly contain one or more bioactive compounds that are more metabolizing than common foods, so, increases the activity of the consumer's body. Due to the health-promoting role of functional foods in the consumers and higher relative prices than other common foods, their monitoring has been vital, and licensing to sell functional food products on the market requires more steps than conventional food products. There are legal requirements and standards for commercial food products, and most manufacturers enter their products in the market following the standards. However, in the case of functional foods in addition to meeting the standards of commercial food products, there should also be defined criteria for assessing the efficiency, bioavailability, and safety of functional food products that contain specified postbiotic components.

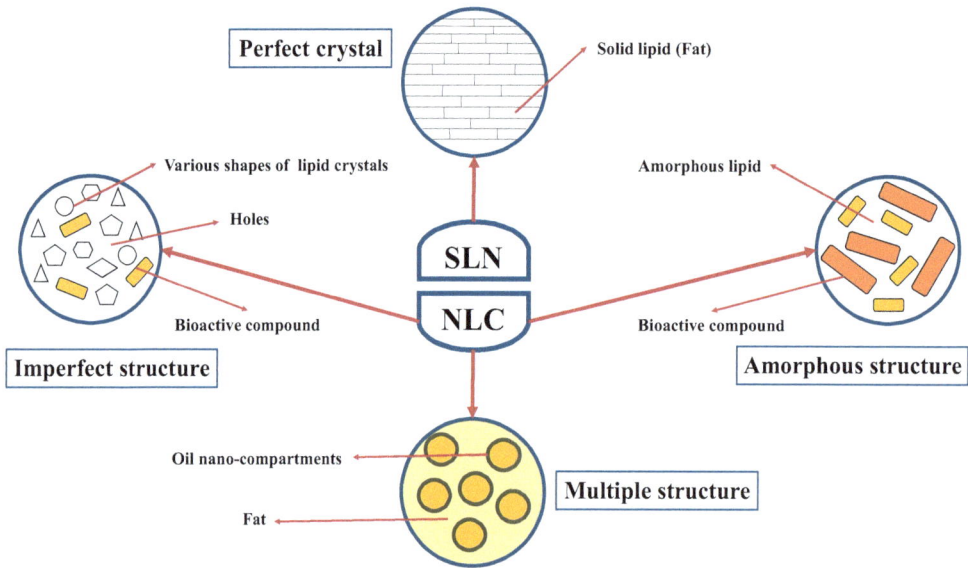

Fig. (8). The structure of SLN and NLC nanocarriers.

Therefore, in order to maintain the health and rights of consumers, it is recommended that the food products with the claim of a particular activity on their labels must go through a series of specialized steps to obtain a commercialization license and enter the market. In this regard, in the case of postbiotic compounds, after identifying the component that possesses a biological activity, to add into the food matrix, its efficiency and stability must first examine in combination with other elements and the processing conditions of carrier food [380]. On the other hand, determining the half-life of the active ingredient (postbiotic compound) to estimate the duration of consumption, checking the effectiveness of the functional food containing postbiotic compounds, and determining the optimal intake in the population and the target group are some of the things that must be observed and controlled by the manufacturer and announced to the competent legal authorities for obtaining a license. The appropriate food carrier for postbiotics is selecting based on the target food characteristics, their production and packaging conditions, as well as the target consumer groups [500].

From a food safety perspective, it is important to evaluate the safety of the postbiotic component alone and along with other components of the food by the manufacturer at the research and development stage. In this regard, the study on the toxicity possibility, immune disorder (food allergy), and the feasibility of consumption by certain groups (infants, children, pregnant women, and vulnerable patients) are the principal indicators for safety approval. Licensing authorities in addition to reviewing the document provided by the manufacturer, conduct a series of independent studies in the laboratory and in the target groups to monitor the safety and effectiveness of the product. Based on the positive results of research conducted by manufacturers and competent authorities, as well as the implementation of various stages of monitoring the nutritional claims of postbiotic functional foods, it is possible to assure the consumer that consuming postbiotic foods in the recommended amount and period will improve your health.

CONCLUSION

Inappropriate lifestyle, increased prevalence of infectious and non-infectious diseases, high treatment costs, adverse effects of some treatment methods, particularly in the treatment of chronic diseases such as cancer, and pay attention to the need for prevention before treatment, including main factors that drive people to change their lifestyle and also to improve their diet. In this regard, nutritionists and food safety experts recommend consuming functional foods, which in addition to meeting the basic nutritional needs, can improve people's health status. On the other hand, along with increasing consumer awareness and subsequently increased research in the functional food field, today new concept has emerged in this field that has excited many research challenges. The evidence from laboratory and clinical studies suggests that postbiotics are safe and have significant efficacy in clinical cases for both prevention and complementary treatment strategies. Postbiotics can describe as biological and functional components of probiotics, which due to their unique functionality, can use in the matrix of a wide range of fermented and non-fermented foods. However, the challenge is to identify new postbiotics and adding them into the food matrix so that they can maintain their biological properties during the production, storage, and preparation process, also determining the appropriate dose of each of the postbiotic compounds for each of their health effects in consumers are among the items that need further research in this field.

REFERENCES

[1]   Hillman ET, Lu H, Yao T, Nakatsu CH. Microbial ecology along the gastrointestinal tract. Microbes Environ 2017; 32(4): 300-13.
[http://dx.doi.org/ 10.1264/jsme2.ME17017] [PMID: 29129876]

[2]   Gholizadeh P, Mahallei M, Pormohammad A, *et al.* Microbial balance in the intestinal microbiota and its association with diabetes, obesity and allergic disease. Microb Pathog 2019; 127: 48-55.
[http://dx.doi.org/ 10.1016/j.micpath.2018.11.031] [PMID: 30503960]

[3]   Subramanian S, Huq S, Yatsunenko T, *et al.* Persistent gut microbiota immaturity in malnourished Bangladeshi children. Nature 2014; 510(7505): 417-21.
[http://dx.doi.org/ 10.1038/nature13421] [PMID: 24896187]

[4]   Presterl E, Diab-El Schahawi M, Lusignani LS, Paula H, Reilly JS. Gastroenteritis: Gastrointestinal Infections. Basic Microbiology and Infection Control for Midwives. Springer 2019; pp. 131-41.
[http://dx.doi.org/ 10.1007/978-3-030-02026-2_14]

[5]   Homayoni Rad A, Akbarzadeh F, Mehrabany EV. Which are more important: prebiotics or probiotics? Nutrition 2012; 28(11-12): 1196-7.
[http://dx.doi.org/ 10.1016/j.nut.2012.03.017] [PMID: 22840387]

[6]   Gholizadeh P, Eslami H, Yousefi M, Asgharzadeh M, Aghazadeh M, Kafil HS. Role of oral microbiome on oral cancers, a review. Biomed Pharmacother 2016; 84: 552-8.
[http://dx.doi.org/ 10.1016/j.biopha.2016.09.082] [PMID: 27693964]

[7]   Hoang TK, He B, Wang T, Tran DQ, Rhoads JM, Liu Y. Protective effect of *Lactobacillus reuteri* DSM 17938 against experimental necrotizing enterocolitis is mediated by Toll-like receptor 2. Am J Physiol Gastrointest Liver Physiol 2018; 315(2): G231-40.
[http://dx.doi.org/ 10.1152/ajpgi.00084.2017] [PMID: 29648878]

[8]   Graspeuntner S, Waschina S, Künzel S, *et al.* Gut dysbiosis with Bacilli dominance and accumulation of fermentation products precedes late-onset sepsis in preterm infants. Clin Infect Dis 2019; 69(2): 268-77.
[http://dx.doi.org/ 10.1093/cid/ciy882] [PMID: 30329017]

[9]   Le Doare K, Holder B, Bassett A, Pannaraj PS. Mother's milk: a purposeful contribution to the development of the infant microbiota and immunity. Front Immunol 2018; 9: 361.
[http://dx.doi.org/ 10.3389/fimmu.2018.00361] [PMID: 29599768]

[10]   Fouhy F, Ross RP, Fitzgerald GF, Stanton C, Cotter PD. Composition of the early intestinal microbiota: knowledge, knowledge gaps and the use of high-throughput sequencing to address these gaps. Gut Microbes 2012; 3(3): 203-20.
[http://dx.doi.org/ 10.4161/gmic.20169] [PMID: 22572829]

[11]   Nagpal R, Mainali R, Ahmadi S, *et al.* Gut microbiome and aging: Physiological and mechanistic insights. Nutr Healthy Aging 2018; 4(4): 267-85.
[http://dx.doi.org/ 10.3233/NHA-170030] [PMID: 29951588]

[12]   Gholizadeh P, Eslami H, Kafil HS. Carcinogenesis mechanisms of *Fusobacterium nucleatum*. Biomed Pharmacother 2017; 89: 918.925
[http://dx.doi.org/ 10.1016/j.biopha.2017.02.102]

[13]   Moludi J, Alizadeh M, Lotfi Yagin N, *et al.* New insights on atherosclerosis: A cross-talk between endocannabinoid systems with gut microbiota. J Cardiovasc Thorac Res 2018; 10(3): 129-37.
[http://dx.doi.org/ 10.15171/jcvtr.2018.21] [PMID: 30386532]

[14]   Schmidt EKA, Torres-Espin A, Raposo PJF, *et al.* Fecal transplant prevents gut dysbiosis and anxiety-like behaviour after spinal cord injury in rats. PLoS One 2020; 15(1). e0226128.

[http://dx.doi.org/ 10.1371/journal.pone.0226128] [PMID: 31940312]

[15] Kafil HS, Mobarez AM, Moghadam MF, Hashemi ZS, Yousefi M. Gentamicin induces efaA expression and biofilm formation in *Enterococcus faecalis*. Microb Pathog 2016; 92: 30-5.
[http://dx.doi.org/ 10.1016/j.micpath.2015.12.008] [PMID: 26724739]

[16] Mortazavi M, Abbasi A, Khodadadi E. Knowledge of parents and status of dental health in children at risk of infective endocarditis. J Dent Shiraz Univ Med Sci 2005; 6(1): 2.

[17] Jabbari V, Khiabani MS, Mokarram RR, *et al.* *Lactobacillus plantarum* as a Probiotic Potential from Kouzeh Cheese (Traditional Iranian Cheese) and Its Antimicrobial Activity. Probiotics Antimicrob Proteins 2017; 9(2): 189-93.
[http://dx.doi.org/ 10.1007/s12602-017-9255-0] [PMID: 28155128]

[18] Homayouni Rad A, Aghebati Maleki L, Samadi Kafil H, Fathi Zavoshti H, Abbasi A. Postbiotics as novel health-promoting ingredients in functional foods. Health Promot Perspect 2020; 10(1): 3-4.
[http://dx.doi.org/ 10.15171/hpp.2020.02] [PMID: 32104650]

[19] Hill C, Guarner F, Reid G, *et al.* Expert consensus document. The International Scientific Association for Probiotics and Prebiotics consensus statement on the scope and appropriate use of the term probiotic. Nat Rev Gastroenterol Hepatol 2014; 11(8): 506-14.
[http://dx.doi.org/ 10.1038/nrgastro.2014.66] [PMID: 24912386]

[20] Anukam KC, Reid G. Probiotics: 100 years (1907–2007) after Elie Metchnikoff's observation. Communicating current research and educational topics and trends in applied microbiology 2007; 1: 466-74.

[21] Abbasi A, Aghebati-Maleki A, Yousefi M, Aghebati-Maleki L. Probiotic intervention as a potential therapeutic for managing gestational disorders and improving pregnancy outcomes. J Reprod Immunol 2021; 143: 103244.
[http://dx.doi.org/ 10.1016/j.jri.2020.103244] [PMID: 33186834]

[22] Jabbari V, *et al.* Molecular Identification of *Lactobacillus acidophilus* as a probiotic potential from traditional doogh samples and evaluation of their antimicrobial activity against some pathogenic bacteria. Biomed Res 2017; 28(4): 1458-63.

[23] Goldenberg J Z, *et al.* Probiotics for the prevention of Clostridium difficile associated diarrhea in adults and children 2017.
[http://dx.doi.org/ 10.1002/14651858.CD006095.pub4]

[24] Shaaban SY, El Gendy YG, Mehanna NS, *et al.* The role of probiotics in children with autism spectrum disorder: A prospective, open-label study. Nutr Neurosci 2018; 21(9): 676-81.
[http://dx.doi.org/ 10.1080/1028415X.2017.1347746] [PMID: 28686541]

[25] Mennini M, Dahdah L, Artesani MC, Fiocchi A, Martelli A. Probiotics in asthma and allergy prevention. Front Pediatr 2017; 5: 165.
[http://dx.doi.org/ 10.3389/fped.2017.00165] [PMID: 28824889]

[26] Zawistowska-Rojek A, Tyski S. Are probiotic really safe for humans? Pol J Microbiol 2018; 67(3): 251-8.
[http://dx.doi.org/ 10.21307/pjm-2018-044] [PMID: 30451441]

[27] Thakur N, Rokana N, Panwar H. Probiotics, Selection criteria, safety and role in health Journal of Innovative Biology 2016; 3(1): 259-70.

[28] Bron PA, Kleerebezem M, Brummer RJ, *et al.* Can probiotics modulate human disease by impacting intestinal barrier function? Br J Nutr 2017; 117(1): 93-107.
[http://dx.doi.org/ 10.1017/S0007114516004037] [PMID: 28102115]

[29] La Fata G, Weber P, Mohajeri MH. Probiotics and the gut immune system: indirect regulation. Probiotics Antimicrob Proteins 2018; 10(1): 11-21.
[http://dx.doi.org/ 10.1007/s12602-017-9322-6] [PMID: 28861741]

[30] Music M, *et al.* Adherence of prebiotic fibers, antioxidants and B complex vitamins on the survival of probiotics. Periodicals of Engineering and Natural Sciences 2020; 8(1): 552-61.

[31] Desrouillères K, Millette M, Bagheri L, Maherani B, Jamshidian M, Lacroix M. The synergistic effect of cell wall extracted from probiotic biomass containing *Lactobacillus acidophilus* CL1285, L. casei LBC80R, and L. rhamnosus CLR2 on the anticancer activity of cranberry juice-HPLC fractions. J Food Biochem 2020; 44(5): e13195.
[http://dx.doi.org/ 10.1111/jfbc.13195] [PMID: 32185816]

[32] Fu L, Cherayil BJ, Shi H, Wang Y, Zhu Y. Food Allergy and the microbiota: implications for probiotic use in regulating allergic responses. Food allergy. Springer 2019; pp. 179-94.
[http://dx.doi.org/ 10.1007/978-981-13-6928-5_8]

[33] Ngongang EFT, *et al.* Effects of probiotic bacteria from yogurt on enzyme and serum cholesterol levels of experimentally induced hyperlipidemic Wistar Albino rats. Am J Biol Life Sci 2016; 4: 48.

[34] Maldonado Galdeano C, Cazorla SI, Lemme Dumit JM, Vélez E, Perdigón G. Beneficial effects of probiotic consumption on the immune system. Ann Nutr Metab 2019; 74(2): 115-24.
[http://dx.doi.org/ 10.1159/000496426] [PMID: 30673668]

[35] Gingold-Belfer R, Levy S, Layfer O, *et al.* Use of a Novel Probiotic Formulation to Alleviate Lactose Intolerance Symptoms-a Pilot Study. Probiotics Antimicrob Proteins 2020; 12(1): 112-8.
[http://dx.doi.org/ 10.1007/s12602-018-9507-7] [PMID: 30617948]

[36] Sánchez B, Delgado S, Blanco-Míguez A, Lourenço A, Gueimonde M, Margolles A. Probiotics, gut microbiota, and their influence on host health and disease. Mol Nutr Food Res 2017; 61(1): 1600240.
[http://dx.doi.org/ 10.1002/mnfr.201600240] [PMID: 27500859]

[37] Zhang P, *et al.* Probiotic mixture ameliorates heat stress of laying hens by enhancing intestinal barrier function and improving gut microbiota. Ital J Anim Sci 2017; 16(2): 292-300.
[http://dx.doi.org/ 10.1080/1828051X.2016.1264261]

[38] Karimi N, Jabbari V, Nazemi A, *et al.* Thymol, cardamom and *Lactobacillus plantarum* nanoparticles as a functional candy with high protection against Streptococcus mutans and tooth decay. Microb Pathog 2020; 148: 104481.
[http://dx.doi.org/ 10.1016/j.micpath.2020.104481] [PMID: 32916244]

[39] Ford AC, Quigley EM, Lacy BE, *et al.* Efficacy of prebiotics, probiotics, and synbiotics in irritable bowel syndrome and chronic idiopathic constipation: systematic review and meta-analysis. Am J Gastroenterol 2014; 109(10): 1547-61.
[http://dx.doi.org/ 10.1038/ajg.2014.202] [PMID: 25070051]

[40] Sahhaf Ebrahimi F, Homayouni Rad A, Mosen M, Abbasalizadeh F, Tabrizi A, Khalili L. Effect of *L. acidophilus* and *B. lactis* on blood glucose in women with gestational diabetes mellitus: a randomized placebo-controlled trial. Diabetol Metab Syndr 2019; 11(1): 75.
[http://dx.doi.org/ 10.1186/s13098-019-0471-5] [PMID: 31485272]

[41] Khalili L, Alipour B, Asghari Jafarabadi M, Hassanalilou T, Mesgari Abbasi M, Faraji I. Probiotic assisted weight management as a main factor for glycemic control in patients with type 2 diabetes: a randomized controlled trial. Diabetol Metab Syndr 2019; 11(1): 5.
[http://dx.doi.org/ 10.1186/s13098-019-0400-7] [PMID: 30675190]

[42] Thomas CM, Versalovic J. Probiotics-host communication: Modulation of signaling pathways in the intestine. Gut Microbes 2010; 1(3): 148-63.
[http://dx.doi.org/ 10.4161/gmic.1.3.11712] [PMID: 20672012]

[43] Hou Q, Zhao F, Liu W, *et al.* Probiotic-directed modulation of gut microbiota is basal microbiome dependent. Gut Microbes 2020; 12(1): 1736974.
[http://dx.doi.org/ 10.1080/19490976.2020.1736974] [PMID: 32200683]

[44] Kristensen NB, Bryrup T, Allin KH, Nielsen T, Hansen TH, Pedersen O. Alterations in fecal microbiota composition by probiotic supplementation in healthy adults: a systematic review of

randomized controlled trials. Genome Med 2016; 8(1): 52.
[http://dx.doi.org/ 10.1186/s13073-016-0300-5] [PMID: 27159972]

[45] Tilg H, Kaser A. Gut microbiome, obesity, and metabolic dysfunction. J Clin Invest 2011; 121(6): 2126-32.
[http://dx.doi.org/ 10.1172/JCI58109] [PMID: 21633181]

[46] Fallucca F, Porrata C, Fallucca S, Pianesi M. Influence of diet on gut microbiota, inflammation and type 2 diabetes mellitus. First experience with macrobiotic Ma-Pi 2 diet. Diabetes Metab Res Rev 2014; 30(S1) (Suppl. 1): 48-54.
[http://dx.doi.org/ 10.1002/dmrr.2518] [PMID: 24532292]

[47] Rad H, Aziz HSK, Zavoshti HF, Shahbazi N, Abbasi A. Therapeutically effects of functional postbiotic foods. Clinical Excellence 2020; 10(2): 33-52.

[48] Metchnikoff E. The prolongation of life: optimistic studies. New York: GP Putnam's Sons 1907.

[49] Pflughoeft KJ, Versalovic J. Human microbiome in health and disease. Annu Rev Pathol 2012; 7: 99-122.
[http://dx.doi.org/ 10.1146/annurev-pathol-011811-132421] [PMID: 21910623]

[50] Frank DN, Zhu W, Sartor RB, Li E. Investigating the biological and clinical significance of human dysbioses. Trends Microbiol 2011; 19(9): 427-34.
[http://dx.doi.org/ 10.1016/j.tim.2011.06.005] [PMID: 21775143]

[51] Cani PD, Delzenne NM. Interplay between obesity and associated metabolic disorders: new insights into the gut microbiota. Curr Opin Pharmacol 2009; 9(6): 737-43.
[http://dx.doi.org/ 10.1016/j.coph.2009.06.016] [PMID: 19628432]

[52] Jumpertz R, Le DS, Turnbaugh PJ, *et al.* Energy-balance studies reveal associations between gut microbes, caloric load, and nutrient absorption in humans. Am J Clin Nutr 2011; 94(1): 58-65.
[http://dx.doi.org/ 10.3945/ajcn.110.010132] [PMID: 21543530]

[53] Preidis GA, Versalovic J. Targeting the human microbiome with antibiotics, probiotics, and prebiotics: gastroenterology enters the metagenomics era. Gastroenterology 2009; 136(6): 2015-31.
[http://dx.doi.org/ 10.1053/j.gastro.2009.01.072] [PMID: 19462507]

[54] Homayouni Rad A, Aghebati Maleki L, Samadi Kafil H, Fathi Zavoshti H, Abbasi A. Postbiotics as Promising Tools for Cancer Adjuvant Therapy. Adv Pharm Bull 2021; 11(1): 1-5.
[http://dx.doi.org/ 10.34172/apb.2021.007] [PMID: 33747846]

[55] Hemarajata P, Versalovic J. Effects of probiotics on gut microbiota: mechanisms of intestinal immunomodulation and neuromodulation. Therap Adv Gastroenterol 2013; 6(1): 39-51.
[http://dx.doi.org/ 10.1177/1756283X12459294] [PMID: 23320049]

[56] O'Shea EF, Cotter PD, Stanton C, Ross RP, Hill C. Production of bioactive substances by intestinal bacteria as a basis for explaining probiotic mechanisms: bacteriocins and conjugated linoleic acid. Int J Food Microbiol 2012; 152(3): 189-205.
[http://dx.doi.org/ 10.1016/j.ijfoodmicro.2011.05.025] [PMID: 21742394]

[57] Collado MC, Meriluoto J, Salminen S. Role of commercial probiotic strains against human pathogen adhesion to intestinal mucus. Lett Appl Microbiol 2007; 45(4): 454-60.
[http://dx.doi.org/ 10.1111/j.1472-765X.2007.02212.x] [PMID: 17897389]

[58] Lee BJ, Bak Y-T. Irritable bowel syndrome, gut microbiota and probiotics. J Neurogastroenterol Motil 2011; 17(3): 252-66.
[http://dx.doi.org/ 10.5056/jnm.2011.17.3.252] [PMID: 21860817]

[59] Bron PA, van Baarlen P, Kleerebezem M. Emerging molecular insights into the interaction between probiotics and the host intestinal mucosa. Nat Rev Microbiol 2011; 10(1): 66-78.
[http://dx.doi.org/ 10.1038/nrmicro2690] [PMID: 22101918]

[60] Nobaek S, Johansson M-L, Molin G, Ahrné S, Jeppsson B. Alteration of intestinal microflora is

associated with reduction in abdominal bloating and pain in patients with irritable bowel syndrome. Am J Gastroenterol 2000; 95(5): 1231-8.
[http://dx.doi.org/ 10.1111/j.1572-0241.2000.02015.x] [PMID: 10811333]

[61]   Ki Cha B, Mun Jung S, Hwan Choi C, *et al.* The effect of a multispecies probiotic mixture on the symptoms and fecal microbiota in diarrhea-dominant irritable bowel syndrome: a randomized, double-blind, placebo-controlled trial. J Clin Gastroenterol 2012; 46(3): 220-7.
[http://dx.doi.org/ 10.1097/MCG.0b013e31823712b1] [PMID: 22157240]

[62]   Cox MJ, Huang YJ, Fujimura KE, *et al.* Lactobacillus casei abundance is associated with profound shifts in the infant gut microbiome. PLoS One 2010; 5(1): e8745.
[http://dx.doi.org/ 10.1371/journal.pone.0008745] [PMID: 20090909]

[63]   Preidis GA, Saulnier DM, Blutt SE, *et al.* Probiotics stimulate enterocyte migration and microbial diversity in the neonatal mouse intestine. FASEB J 2012; 26(5): 1960-9.
[http://dx.doi.org/ 10.1096/fj.10-177980] [PMID: 22267340]

[64]   Eisenhauer N, Scheu S, Jousset A. Bacterial diversity stabilizes community productivity. PLoS One 2012; 7(3): e34517.
[http://dx.doi.org/ 10.1371/journal.pone.0034517] [PMID: 22470577]

[65]   McNulty NP, *et al.* The impact of a consortium of fermented milk strains on the gut microbiome of gnotobiotic mice and monozygotic twins. 2011.
[http://dx.doi.org/ 10.1126/scitranslmed.3002701]

[66]   Furness JB. Novel gut afferents: Intrinsic afferent neurons and intestinofugal neurons. Auton Neurosci 2006; 125(1-2): 81-5.
[http://dx.doi.org/ 10.1016/j.autneu.2006.01.007] [PMID: 16476573]

[67]   Grenham S, Clarke G, Cryan JF, Dinan TG. Brain-gut-microbe communication in health and disease. Front Physiol 2011; 2: 94.
[http://dx.doi.org/ 10.3389/fphys.2011.00094] [PMID: 22162969]

[68]   Tabrizi A, Khalili L, Homayouni-Rad A, Pourjafar H, Dehghan P, Ansari F. Prebiotics, as Promising Functional Food to Patients with Psychological Disorders: A Review on Mood Disorders, Sleep, and Cognition. Neuroquantology 2019; 17(6)
[http://dx.doi.org/ 10.14704/nq.2019.17.6.2189]

[69]   Cryan JF, Dinan TG. Mind-altering microorganisms: the impact of the gut microbiota on brain and behaviour. Nat Rev Neurosci 2012; 13(10): 701-12.
[http://dx.doi.org/ 10.1038/nrn3346] [PMID: 22968153]

[70]   Neufeld KM, Kang N, Bienenstock J, Foster JA. Reduced anxiety-like behavior and central neurochemical change in germ-free mice. Neurogastroenterol Motil 2011; 23(3): 255-264, e119.
[http://dx.doi.org/ 10.1111/j.1365-2982.2010.01620.x] [PMID: 21054680]

[71]   Gareau MG, Wine E, Rodrigues DM, *et al.* Bacterial infection causes stress-induced memory dysfunction in mice. Gut 2011; 60(3): 307-17.
[http://dx.doi.org/ 10.1136/gut.2009.202515] [PMID: 20966022]

[72]   Dinan TG, Cryan JF. Melancholic microbes: a link between gut microbiota and depression? Neurogastroenterol Motil 2013; 25(9): 713-9.
[http://dx.doi.org/ 10.1111/nmo.12198] [PMID: 23910373]

[73]   Moloney RD, Desbonnet L, Clarke G, Dinan TG, Cryan JF. The microbiome: stress, health and disease. Mamm Genome 2014; 25(1-2): 49-74.
[http://dx.doi.org/ 10.1007/s00335-013-9488-5] [PMID: 24281320]

[74]   Hardy H, Harris J, Lyon E, Beal J, Foey AD. Probiotics, prebiotics and immunomodulation of gut mucosal defences: homeostasis and immunopathology. Nutrients 2013; 5(6): 1869-912.
[http://dx.doi.org/ 10.3390/nu5061869] [PMID: 23760057]

[75]   Tillisch K, *et al.* Consumption of fermented milk product with probiotic modulates brain activity.

2013.
[http://dx.doi.org/ 10.1053/j.gastro.2013.02.043]

[76] Shi Y, Liu J, Yan Q, You X, Yang S, Jiang Z. *In vitro* digestibility and prebiotic potential of curdlan (1 → 3)-β-d-glucan oligosaccharides in Lactobacillus species. Carbohydr Polym 2018; 188: 17-26.
[http://dx.doi.org/ 10.1016/j.carbpol.2018.01.085] [PMID: 29525154]

[77] Ahmadi S, Nagpal R, Wang S, *et al.* Prebiotics from acorn and sago prevent high-fat-diet-induced insulin resistance *via* microbiome-gut-brain axis modulation. J Nutr Biochem 2019; 67: 1-13.
[http://dx.doi.org/ 10.1016/j.jnutbio.2019.01.011] [PMID: 30831458]

[78] Subramanian VS, Sabui S, Heskett CW, Said HM. Sodium butyrate enhances intestinal riboflavin uptake *via* induction of expression of riboflavin transporter-3 (RFVT3). Dig Dis Sci 2019; 64(1): 84-92.
[http://dx.doi.org/ 10.1007/s10620-018-5305-z] [PMID: 30276569]

[79] Verma DK, Niamah AK, Patel AR, *et al.* Chemistry and microbial sources of curdlan with potential application and safety regulations as prebiotic in food and health. Food Res Int 2020; 133: 109136.
[http://dx.doi.org/ 10.1016/j.foodres.2020.109136] [PMID: 32466929]

[80] Ghanbari M, Saeedi M, Mortazavian AM. Nutraceuticals and Functional Foods production. Clinical Excellence 2016; 5(1): 1-15.

[81] Maeda-Yamamoto M. Development of functional agricultural products and use of a new health claim system in Japan. Trends Food Sci Technol 2017; 69: 324-32.
[http://dx.doi.org/ 10.1016/j.tifs.2017.08.011]

[82] Shimizu T. Health claims and scientific substantiation of functional foods-Japanese system aiming the global standard. Curr Top Nutraceutical Res 2003; 1: 213-24.

[83] Meybodi N M, Mortazavian A M, Sohrabvandi S, Cruz A G D, Mohammadi Reza. Probiotic supplements and food products: comparison for different targets Applied Food Biotechnology 2017; 4(3): 123-32.

[84] Shahidi F. Functional foods: their role in health promotion and disease prevention. J Food Sci 2004; 69(5): R146-9.
[http://dx.doi.org/ 10.1111/j.1365-2621.2004.tb10727.x]

[85] Min M, Bunt CR, Mason SL, Hussain MA. Non-dairy probiotic food products: An emerging group of functional foods. Crit Rev Food Sci Nutr 2019; 59(16): 2626-41.
[http://dx.doi.org/ 10.1080/10408398.2018.1462760] [PMID: 29630845]

[86] Aguilar-Toalá J, *et al.* Postbiotics: An evolving term within the functional foods field. Trends Food Sci Technol 2018; 75: 105-14.
[http://dx.doi.org/ 10.1016/j.tifs.2018.03.009]

[87] Homayouni Rad A, Aghebati Maleki L, Samadi Kafil H, Abbasi A. Postbiotics: A novel strategy in food allergy treatment. Crit Rev Food Sci Nutr 2020; 1-8.
[http://dx.doi.org/ 10.1080/10408398.2020.1738333] [PMID: 32160762]

[88] Boyle RJ, Robins-Browne RM, Tang ML. Probiotic use in clinical practice: what are the risks? Am J Clin Nutr 2006; 83(6): 1256-64.
[http://dx.doi.org/ 10.1093/ajcn/83.6.1256] [PMID: 16762934]

[89] Jalili H, Razavi H, Safari M, Amrane A. Kinetic analysis and effect of culture medium and coating materials during free and immobilized cell cultures of *Bifidobacterium* animalis subsp. lactis Bb 12. Electron J Biotechnol 2010; 13(3): 2-3.
[http://dx.doi.org/ 10.2225/vol13-issue3-fulltext-4]

[90] Akbarian-rad Z, Zahedpasha Y, Ahmadpour-kacho M, Taghipour Y. The effect of probiotic lactobacillus reuteri on reducing the period of restlessness in infants with colic. Majallah-i Danishgah-i Ulum-i Pizishki-i Babul 2015; 17(5): 7-11.

[91]   Kaila M, Isolauri E, Saxelin M, Arvilommi H, Vesikari T. Viable *versus* inactivated *Lactobacillus strain* GG in acute rotavirus diarrhoea. Arch Dis Child 1995; 72(1): 51-3.
       [http://dx.doi.org/ 10.1136/adc.72.1.51] [PMID: 7717739]

[92]   Abney KN, Hewlings SJ. Probiotic supplementation and reducing infiammation in hemodialysis patients: A systematic review. Journal of Renal Nutrition and Metabolism 2019; 5(1): 3.
       [http://dx.doi.org/ 10.4103/jrnm.jrnm_16_19]

[93]   Theunissen J, Britz TJ, Torriani S, Witthuhn RC. Identification of probiotic microorganisms in South African products using PCR-based DGGE analysis. Int J Food Microbiol 2005; 98(1): 11-21.
       [http://dx.doi.org/ 10.1016/j.ijfoodmicro.2004.05.004] [PMID: 15617797]

[94]   Gezginc Y, Topcal F, Comertpay S, Akyol I. Quantitative analysis of the lactic acid and acetaldehyde produced by Streptococcus thermophilus and Lactobacillus bulgaricus strains isolated from traditional Turkish yogurts using HPLC. J Dairy Sci 2015; 98(3): 1426-34.
       [http://dx.doi.org/ 10.3168/jds.2014-8447] [PMID: 25547312]

[95]   Kaur IP, Chopra K, Saini A. Probiotics: potential pharmaceutical applications. Eur J Pharm Sci 2002; 15(1): 1-9.
       [http://dx.doi.org/ 10.1016/S0928-0987(01)00209-3] [PMID: 11803126]

[96]   Apostolou E, Kirjavainen PV, Saxelin M, *et al.* Good adhesion properties of probiotics: a potential risk for bacteremia? FEMS Immunol Med Microbiol 2001; 31(1): 35-9.
       [http://dx.doi.org/ 10.1111/j.1574-695X.2001.tb01583.x] [PMID: 11476979]

[97]   ten Brink B, Damink C, Joosten HM, Huis in 't Veld JH. Occurrence and formation of biologically active amines in foods. Int J Food Microbiol 1990; 11(1): 73-84.
       [http://dx.doi.org/ 10.1016/0168-1605(90)90040-C] [PMID: 2223522]

[98]   O'Brien J, Crittenden R, Ouwehand AC, Salminen S. Safety evaluation of probiotics. Trends Food Sci Technol 1999; 10(12): 418-24.
       [http://dx.doi.org/ 10.1016/S0924-2244(00)00037-6]

[99]   Cohen PA. Probiotic safety—no guarantees. JAMA Intern Med 2018; 178(12): 1577-8.
       [http://dx.doi.org/ 10.1001/jamainternmed.2018.5403] [PMID: 30242393]

[100]   Doron S, Snydman D R. Risk and safety of probiotics 2015.
       [http://dx.doi.org/ 10.1093/cid/civ085]

[101]   Lherm T, Monet C, Nougière B, *et al.* Seven cases of fungemia with Saccharomyces boulardii in critically ill patients. Intensive Care Med 2002; 28(6): 797-801.
       [http://dx.doi.org/ 10.1007/s00134-002-1267-9] [PMID: 12107689]

[102]   Oggioni MR, Pozzi G, Valensin PE, Galieni P, Bigazzi C. Recurrent septicemia in an immunocompromised patient due to probiotic strains of Bacillus subtilis. J Clin Microbiol 1998; 36(1): 325-6.
       [http://dx.doi.org/ 10.1128/JCM.36.1.325-326.1998] [PMID: 9431982]

[103]   Franz CM, Holzapfel WH, Stiles ME. Enterococci at the crossroads of food safety? Int J Food Microbiol 1999; 47(1-2): 1-24.
       [http://dx.doi.org/ 10.1016/S0168-1605(99)00007-0] [PMID: 10357269]

[104]   Hammes WP, Hertel C. Research approaches for pre-and probiotics: challenges and outlook. Food Res Int 2002; 35(2-3): 165-70.
       [http://dx.doi.org/ 10.1016/S0963-9969(01)00178-8]

[105]   Murray BE. Diversity among multidrug-resistant enterococci. Emerg Infect Dis 1998; 4(1): 37-47.
       [http://dx.doi.org/ 10.3201/eid0401.980106] [PMID: 9452397]

[106]   Borriello SP, Hammes WP, Holzapfel W, *et al.* Safety of probiotics that contain lactobacilli or bifidobactcria. Clin Infect Dis 2003; 36(6): 775-80.
       [http://dx.doi.org/ 10.1086/368080] [PMID: 12627362]

[107] Cannon JP, Lee TA, Bolanos JT, Danziger LH. Pathogenic relevance of Lactobacillus: a retrospective review of over 200 cases. Eur J Clin Microbiol Infect Dis 2005; 24(1): 31-40.
[http://dx.doi.org/ 10.1007/s10096-004-1253-y] [PMID: 15599646]

[108] Rautio M, Jousimies-Somer H, Kauma H, *et al.* Liver abscess due to a *Lactobacillus rhamnosus* strain indistinguishable from L. rhamnosus strain GG. Clin Infect Dis 1999; 28(5): 1159-60.
[http://dx.doi.org/ 10.1086/514766] [PMID: 10452653]

[109] Pochard P, Gosset P, Grangette C, *et al.* Lactic acid bacteria inhibit TH2 cytokine production by mononuclear cells from allergic patients. J Allergy Clin Immunol 2002; 110(4): 617-23.
[http://dx.doi.org/ 10.1067/mai.2002.128528] [PMID: 12373271]

[110] Mackay AD, Taylor MB, Kibbler CC, Hamilton-Miller JM. *Lactobacillus endocarditis* caused by a probiotic organism. Clin Microbiol Infect 1999; 5(5): 290-2.
[http://dx.doi.org/ 10.1111/j.1469-0691.1999.tb00144.x] [PMID: 11856270]

[111] Kunz AN, Noel JM, Fairchok MP. Two cases of *Lactobacillus bacteremia* during probiotic treatment of short gut syndrome. J Pediatr Gastroenterol Nutr 2004; 38(4): 457-8.
[http://dx.doi.org/ 10.1097/00005176-200404000-00017] [PMID: 15085028]

[112] De Groote MA, Frank DN, Dowell E, Glode MP, Pace NR. *Lactobacillus rhamnosus* GG bacteremia associated with probiotic use in a child with short gut syndrome. Pediatr Infect Dis J 2005; 24(3): 278-80.
[http://dx.doi.org/ 10.1097/01.inf.0000154588.79356.e6] [PMID: 15750472]

[113] Dani C, Coviello C C, Corsini I I, Arena F, Antonelli A, Rossolini GM. *Lactobacillus Sepsis* and Probiotic Therapy in Newborns: Two New Cases and Literature Review. AJP Rep 2016; 6(1): e25-9.
[PMID: 26929865]

[114] Richard V, Van der Auwera P, Snoeck R, Daneau D, Meunier F. Nosocomial bacteremia caused byBacillus species 1988.
[http://dx.doi.org/ 10.1007/BF01975049]

[115] Spinosa MR. The Trouble in Tracing Opportunistic Pathogens: Cholangitis due to Bacillus in a French Hospital Caused by a Strain Related to an Italian Probiotic? Microb Ecol Health Dis 2000; 12(2): 99-101.

[116] Vankerckhoven V, *et al.* Biosafety assessment of probiotics used for human consumption: recommendations from the EU-PROSAFE project. Trends Food Sci Technol 2008; 19(2): 102-14.
[http://dx.doi.org/ 10.1016/j.tifs.2007.07.013]

[117] Nicas TI, Cole CT, Preston DA, Schabel AA, Nagarajan R. Activity of glycopeptides against vancomycin-resistant gram-positive bacteria. Antimicrob Agents Chemother 1989; 33(9): 1477-81.
[http://dx.doi.org/ 10.1128/AAC.33.9.1477] [PMID: 2817848]

[118] Swenson JM, Facklam RR, Thornsberry C. Antimicrobial susceptibility of vancomycin-resistant Leuconostoc, Pediococcus, and Lactobacillus species. Antimicrob Agents Chemother 1990; 34(4): 543-9.
[http://dx.doi.org/ 10.1128/AAC.34.4.543] [PMID: 2344161]

[119] Billot-Klein D, Gutmann L, Sablé S, Guittet E, van Heijenoort J. Modification of peptidoglycan precursors is a common feature of the low-level vancomycin-resistant VANB-type Enterococcus D366 and of the naturally glycopeptide-resistant species *Lactobacillus casei*, *Pediococcus pentosaceus*, *Leuconostoc mesenteroides*, and *Enterococcus gallinarum*. J Bacteriol 1994; 176(8): 2398-405.
[http://dx.doi.org/ 10.1128/JB.176.8.2398-2405.1994] [PMID: 8157610]

[120] Saarela M, Mogensen G, Fondén R, Mättö J, Mattila-Sandholm T. Probiotic bacteria: safety, functional and technological properties. J Biotechnol 2000; 84(3): 197-215.
[http://dx.doi.org/ 10.1016/S0168-1656(00)00375-8] [PMID: 11164262]

[121] Courvalin P. Transfer of antibiotic resistance genes between gram-positive and gram-negative bacteria. Antimicrob Agents Chemother 1994; 38(7): 1447-51.

[http://dx.doi.org/ 10.1128/AAC.38.7.1447] [PMID: 7979269]

[122] Moubareck C, Gavini F, Vaugien L, Butel MJ, Doucet-Populaire F. Antimicrobial susceptibility of bifidobacteria. J Antimicrob Chemother 2005; 55(1): 38-44.
[http://dx.doi.org/ 10.1093/jac/dkh495] [PMID: 15574479]

[123] Muñoz-Atienza E, Landeta G, de las Rivas B, *et al.* Phenotypic and genetic evaluations of biogenic amine production by lactic acid bacteria isolated from fish and fish products. Int J Food Microbiol 2011; 146(2): 212-6.
[http://dx.doi.org/ 10.1016/j.ijfoodmicro.2011.02.024] [PMID: 21411165]

[124] Halász A, Baráth Á, Simon-Sarkadi L, Holzapfel W. Biogenic amines and their production by microorganisms in food. Trends Food Sci Technol 1994; 5(2): 42-9.
[http://dx.doi.org/ 10.1016/0924-2244(94)90070-1]

[125] Ammor MS, Mayo B. Selection criteria for lactic acid bacteria to be used as functional starter cultures in dry sausage production: An update. Meat Sci 2007; 76(1): 138-46.
[http://dx.doi.org/ 10.1016/j.meatsci.2006.10.022] [PMID: 22064200]

[126] Stadnik J, Dolatowski ZJ. Biogenic amines content during extended ageing of dry-cured pork loins inoculated with probiotics. Meat Sci 2012; 91(3): 374-7.
[http://dx.doi.org/ 10.1016/j.meatsci.2012.02.022] [PMID: 22417730]

[127] da Cruz AG, Buriti FCA, de Souza CHB, Faria JAF, Saad SMI. Probiotic cheese: health benefits, technological and stability aspects. Trends Food Sci Technol 2009; 20(8): 344-54.
[http://dx.doi.org/ 10.1016/j.tifs.2009.05.001]

[128] Mattila-Sandholm T, Myllärinen P, Crittenden R, Mogensen G, Fondén R, Saarela M. Technological challenges for future probiotic foods. Int Dairy J 2002; 12(2-3): 173-82.
[http://dx.doi.org/ 10.1016/S0958-6946(01)00099-1]

[129] Evivie SE, Huo G-C, Igene JO, Bian X. Some current applications, limitations and future perspectives of lactic acid bacteria as probiotics. Food Nutr Res 2017; 61(1): 1318034.
[http://dx.doi.org/ 10.1080/16546628.2017.1318034] [PMID: 28659729]

[130] Evivie S. Preliminary studies on pharmaceutical microencapsulation for synbiotic application. J Appl Nat Sci 2013; 5(2): 488-96.
[http://dx.doi.org/ 10.31018/jans.v5i2.358]

[131] Nakai M, Okahashi N, Ohta H, Koga T. Saliva-binding region of Streptococcus mutans surface protein antigen. Infect Immun 1993; 61(10): 4344-9.
[http://dx.doi.org/ 10.1128/IAI.61.10.4344-4349.1993] [PMID: 8406823]

[132] Wagner RD, Warner T, Roberts L, Farmer J, Balish E. Colonization of congenitally immunodeficient mice with probiotic bacteria. Infect Immun 1997; 65(8): 3345-51.
[http://dx.doi.org/ 10.1128/IAI.65.8.3345-3351.1997] [PMID: 9234796]

[133] de Almada CN, Almada CN, Martinez RC, Sant'Ana AS. Paraprobiotics: evidences on their ability to modify biological responses, inactivation methods and perspectives on their application in foods. Trends Food Sci Technol 2016; 58: 96-114.
[http://dx.doi.org/ 10.1016/j.tifs.2016.09.011]

[134] Barros CP, *et al.* Paraprobiotics and postbiotics: Concepts and potential applications in dairy products. Curr Opin Food Sci 2020; 32: 1-8.
[http://dx.doi.org/ 10.1016/j.cofs.2019.12.003]

[135] Engevik MA, Versalovic J. Biochemical features of beneficial microbes: foundations for therapeutic microbiology. Bugs as Drugs: Therapeutic Microbes for the Prevention and Treatment of Disease 2018; 1-47.

[136] Singh A, Vishwakarma V, Singhal B. Metabiotics: the functional metabolic signatures of probiotics: current state-of-art and future research priorities—metabiotics: probiotics effector molecules. Adv Biosci Biotechnol 2018; 9(4): 147-89.

[http://dx.doi.org/ 10.4236/abb.2018.94012]

[137] Levy M, Kolodziejczyk AA, Thaiss CA, Elinav E. Dysbiosis and the immune system. Nat Rev Immunol 2017; 17(4): 219-32.
[http://dx.doi.org/ 10.1038/nri.2017.7] [PMID: 28260787]

[138] Thaiss CA, Elinav E. The remedy within: will the microbiome fulfill its therapeutic promise? J Mol Med (Berl) 2017; 95(10): 1021-7.
[http://dx.doi.org/ 10.1007/s00109-017-1563-z] [PMID: 28656322]

[139] Bennett BJ, de Aguiar Vallim TQ, Wang Z, *et al.* Trimethylamine-N-oxide, a metabolite associated with atherosclerosis, exhibits complex genetic and dietary regulation. Cell Metab 2013; 17(1): 49-60.
[http://dx.doi.org/ 10.1016/j.cmet.2012.12.011] [PMID: 23312283]

[140] Tan Y, Sheng Z, Zhou P, *et al.* Plasma trimethylamine N-oxide as a novel biomarker for plaque rupture in patients with ST-segment-elevation myocardial infarction. Circ Cardiovasc Interv 2019; 12(1): e007281.
[http://dx.doi.org/ 10.1161/CIRCINTERVENTIONS.118.007281] [PMID: 30599768]

[141] Zhuang R, Ge X, Han L, *et al.* Gut microbe-generated metabolite trimethylamine N-oxide and the risk of diabetes: A systematic review and dose-response meta-analysis. Obes Rev 2019; 20(6): 883-94.
[http://dx.doi.org/ 10.1111/obr.12843] [PMID: 30868721]

[142] Haghikia A, Li XS, Liman TG, *et al.* Gut microbiota–dependent trimethylamine N-oxide predicts risk of cardiovascular events in patients with stroke and is related to proinflammatory monocytes. Arterioscler Thromb Vasc Biol 2018; 38(9): 2225-35.
[http://dx.doi.org/ 10.1161/ATVBAHA.118.311023] [PMID: 29976769]

[143] Li XS, Wang Z, Cajka T, *et al.* Untargeted metabolomics identifies trimethyllysine, a TMAO-producing nutrient precursor, as a predictor of incident cardiovascular disease risk. JCI Insight 2018; 3(6): 99096.
[http://dx.doi.org/ 10.1172/jci.insight.99096] [PMID: 29563342]

[144] Missailidis C, Hällqvist J, Qureshi AR, *et al.* Serum trimethylamine-N-oxide is strongly related to renal function and predicts outcome in chronic kidney disease. PLoS One 2016; 11(1): e0141738.
[http://dx.doi.org/ 10.1371/journal.pone.0141738] [PMID: 26751065]

[145] Stubbs JR, Stedman MR, Liu S, *et al.* Trimethylamine N-oxide and cardiovascular outcomes in patients with ESKD receiving maintenance hemodialysis. Clin J Am Soc Nephrol 2019; 14(2): 261-7.
[http://dx.doi.org/ 10.2215/CJN.06190518] [PMID: 30665924]

[146] Vogt NM, Romano KA, Darst BF, *et al.* The gut microbiota-derived metabolite trimethylamine N-oxide is elevated in Alzheimer's disease. Alzheimers Res Ther 2018; 10(1): 124.
[http://dx.doi.org/ 10.1186/s13195-018-0451-2] [PMID: 30579367]

[147] Koeth RA, Wang Z, Levison BS, *et al.* Intestinal microbiota metabolism of L-carnitine, a nutrient in red meat, promotes atherosclerosis. Nat Med 2013; 19(5): 576-85.
[http://dx.doi.org/ 10.1038/nm.3145] [PMID: 23563705]

[148] Zhu W, Buffa JA, Wang Z, *et al.* Flavin monooxygenase 3, the host hepatic enzyme in the metaorganismal trimethylamine N-oxide-generating pathway, modulates platelet responsiveness and thrombosis risk. J Thromb Haemost 2018; 16(9): 1857-72.
[http://dx.doi.org/ 10.1111/jth.14234] [PMID: 29981269]

[149] Wang Z, Klipfell E, Bennett BJ, *et al.* Gut flora metabolism of phosphatidylcholine promotes cardiovascular disease. Nature 2011; 472(7341): 57-63.
[http://dx.doi.org/ 10.1038/nature09922] [PMID: 21475195]

[150] Warrier M, Shih DM, Burrows AC, *et al.* The TMAO-generating enzyme flavin monooxygenase 3 is a central regulator of cholesterol balance. Cell Rep 2015; 10(3): 326-38.
[http://dx.doi.org/ 10.1016/j.celrep.2014.12.036] [PMID: 25600868]

[151] Ding L, Chang M, Guo Y, *et al.* Trimethylamine-N-oxide (TMAO)-induced atherosclerosis is

associated with bile acid metabolism. Lipids Health Dis 2018; 17(1): 286.
[http://dx.doi.org/ 10.1186/s12944-018-0939-6] [PMID: 30567573]

[152] Zhu W, Gregory JC, Org E, *et al.* Gut microbial metabolite TMAO enhances platelet hyperreactivity and thrombosis risk. Cell 2016; 165(1): 111-24.
[http://dx.doi.org/ 10.1016/j.cell.2016.02.011] [PMID: 26972052]

[153] Wang Z, Roberts AB, Buffa JA, *et al.* Non-lethal inhibition of gut microbial trimethylamine production for the treatment of atherosclerosis. Cell 2015; 163(7): 1585-95.
[http://dx.doi.org/ 10.1016/j.cell.2015.11.055] [PMID: 26687352]

[154] Velasquez MT, Ramezani A, Manal A, Raj DS. Trimethylamine N-oxide: the good, the bad and the unknown. Toxins (Basel) 2016; 8(11): 326.
[http://dx.doi.org/ 10.3390/toxins8110326] [PMID: 27834801]

[155] Rad AH, Abbasi A, Javadi A, Pourjafar H, Javadi M, Khaleghi M. Comparing the microbial quality of traditional and industrial yoghurts. Biointerface Research in Applied Chemistry 2020; 10(4): 6020-5.
[http://dx.doi.org/ 10.33263/BRIAC104.020025]

[156] Chang PV, Hao L, Offermanns S, Medzhitov R. The microbial metabolite butyrate regulates intestinal macrophage function *via* histone deacetylase inhibition. Proc Natl Acad Sci USA 2014; 111(6): 2247-52.
[http://dx.doi.org/ 10.1073/pnas.1322269111] [PMID: 24390544]

[157] Schulthess J, *et al.* The short chain fatty acid butyrate imprints an antimicrobial program in macrophages. 2019.
[http://dx.doi.org/ 10.1016/j.immuni.2018.12.018]

[158] Sun M, Wu W, Chen L, *et al.* Microbiota-derived short-chain fatty acids promote Th1 cell IL-10 production to maintain intestinal homeostasis. Nat Commun 2018; 9(1): 3555.
[http://dx.doi.org/ 10.1038/s41467-018-05901-2] [PMID: 30177845]

[159] Smith PM, Howitt MR, Panikov N, *et al.* The microbial metabolites, short-chain fatty acids, regulate colonic Treg cell homeostasis. Science 2013; 341(6145): 569-73.
[http://dx.doi.org/ 10.1126/science.1241165] [PMID: 23828891]

[160] Arpaia N, Campbell C, Fan X, *et al.* Metabolites produced by commensal bacteria promote peripheral regulatory T-cell generation. Nature 2013; 504(7480): 451-5.
[http://dx.doi.org/ 10.1038/nature12726] [PMID: 24226773]

[161] Wu W, Sun M, Chen F, *et al.* Microbiota metabolite short-chain fatty acid acetate promotes intestinal IgA response to microbiota which is mediated by GPR43. Mucosal Immunol 2017; 10(4): 946-56.
[http://dx.doi.org/ 10.1038/mi.2016.114] [PMID: 27966553]

[162] Kim M, Friesen L, Park J, Kim HM, Kim CH. Microbial metabolites, short-chain fatty acids, restrain tissue bacterial load, chronic inflammation, and associated cancer in the colon of mice. Eur J Immunol 2018; 48(7): 1235-47.
[http://dx.doi.org/ 10.1002/eji.201747122] [PMID: 29644622]

[163] Kimura I, *et al.* The gut microbiota suppresses insulin-mediated fat accumulation via the short-chain fatty acid receptor GPR43 2013.
[http://dx.doi.org/ 10.1038/ncomms2852]

[164] Yoo D Y, *et al.* Synergistic Effects of Sodium Butyrate, a Histone Deacetylase Inhibitor, on Increase of Neurogenesis Induced by Pyridoxine and Increase of Neural Proliferation in the Mouse Dentate Gyrus 2011.
[http://dx.doi.org/ 10.1007/s11064-011-0503-5]

[165] Slingerland AE, Schwabkey Z, Wiesnoski DH, Jenq RR. Clinical Evidence for the Microbiome in Inflammatory Diseases. 2017.
[http://dx.doi.org/ 10.3389/fimmu.2017.00400]

[166] Puddu A, Sanguineti R, Montecucco F, Viviani GL. Evidence for the Gut Microbiota Short-Chain

Fatty Acids as Key Pathophysiological Molecules Improving Diabetes. 2014.
[http://dx.doi.org/ 10.1155/2014/162021]

[167] Hamer HM, Jonkers DM, Bast A, *et al.* Butyrate modulates oxidative stress in the colonic mucosa of healthy humans. Clin Nutr 2009; 28(1): 88-93.
[http://dx.doi.org/ 10.1016/j.clnu.2008.11.002] [PMID: 19108937]

[168] Cuomo A, Maina G, Rosso G, *et al.* The microbiome: a new target for research and treatment of schizophrenia and its resistant presentations? A systematic literature search and review. Front Pharmacol 2018; 9: 1040.
[http://dx.doi.org/ 10.3389/fphar.2018.01040] [PMID: 30374300]

[169] Erny D, Hrabě de Angelis AL, Jaitin D, *et al.* Host microbiota constantly control maturation and function of microglia in the CNS. Nat Neurosci 2015; 18(7): 965-77.
[http://dx.doi.org/ 10.1038/nn.4030] [PMID: 26030851]

[170] Buffington SA, Di Prisco GV, Auchtung TA, Ajami NJ, Petrosino JF, Costa-Mattioli M. Microbial reconstitution reverses maternal diet-induced social and synaptic deficits in offspring. Cell 2016; 165(7): 1762-75.
[http://dx.doi.org/ 10.1016/j.cell.2016.06.001] [PMID: 27315483]

[171] Bourassa MW, Alim I, Bultman SJ, Ratan RR. Butyrate, neuroepigenetics and the gut microbiome: Can a high fiber diet improve brain health? Neurosci Lett 2016; 625: 56-63.
[http://dx.doi.org/ 10.1016/j.neulet.2016.02.009] [PMID: 26868600]

[172] Govindarajan N, Agis-Balboa RC, Walter J, Sananbenesi F, Fischer A. Sodium butyrate improves memory function in an Alzheimer's disease mouse model when administered at an advanced stage of disease progression. J Alzheimers Dis 2011; 26(1): 187-97.
[http://dx.doi.org/ 10.3233/JAD-2011-110080] [PMID: 21593570]

[173] Lopes-Borges J, Valvassori SS, Varela RB, *et al.* Histone deacetylase inhibitors reverse manic-like behaviors and protect the rat brain from energetic metabolic alterations induced by ouabain. Pharmacol Biochem Behav 2015; 128: 89-95.
[http://dx.doi.org/ 10.1016/j.pbb.2014.11.014] [PMID: 25433326]

[174] Burokas A, Arboleya S, Moloney RD, *et al.* Targeting the microbiota-gut-brain axis: prebiotics have anxiolytic and antidepressant-like effects and reverse the impact of chronic stress in mice. Biol Psychiatry 2017; 82(7): 472-87.
[http://dx.doi.org/ 10.1016/j.biopsych.2016.12.031] [PMID: 28242013]

[175] Shibata N, Kunisawa J, Kiyono H. Dietary and microbial metabolites in the regulation of host immunity. Front Microbiol 2017; 8: 2171.
[http://dx.doi.org/ 10.3389/fmicb.2017.02171] [PMID: 29163449]

[176] Hirata SI, Kunisawa J. Gut microbiome, metabolome, and allergic diseases. Allergol Int 2017; 66(4): 523-8.
[http://dx.doi.org/ 10.1016/j.alit.2017.06.008] [PMID: 28693971]

[177] Kishino S, Takeuchi M, Park SB, *et al.* Polyunsaturated fatty acid saturation by gut lactic acid bacteria affecting host lipid composition. Proc Natl Acad Sci USA 2013; 110(44): 17808-13.
[http://dx.doi.org/ 10.1073/pnas.1312937110] [PMID: 24127592]

[178] Bassaganya-Riera J, Hontecillas R, Horne WT, *et al.* Conjugated linoleic acid modulates immune responses in patients with mild to moderately active Crohn's disease. Clin Nutr 2012; 31(5): 721-7.
[http://dx.doi.org/ 10.1016/j.clnu.2012.03.002] [PMID: 22521469]

[179] Kaikiri H, Miyamoto J, Kawakami T, *et al.* Supplemental feeding of a gut microbial metabolite of linoleic acid, 10-hydroxy-cis-12-octadecenoic acid, alleviates spontaneous atopic dermatitis and modulates intestinal microbiota in NC/nga mice. Int J Food Sci Nutr 2017; 68(8): 941-51.
[http://dx.doi.org/ 10.1080/09637486.2017.1318116] [PMID: 28438083]

[180] Miyamoto J, Mizukure T, Park SB, *et al.* A gut microbial metabolite of linoleic acid, 10-hydroxy-c-

s-12-octadecenoic acid, ameliorates intestinal epithelial barrier impairment partially *via* GPR40-ME-
-ERK pathway. J Biol Chem 2015; 290(5): 2902-18.
[http://dx.doi.org/ 10.1074/jbc.M114.610733] [PMID: 25505251]

[181] Gaullier J-M, Halse J, Høivik HO, *et al*. Six months supplementation with conjugated linoleic acid induces regional-specific fat mass decreases in overweight and obese. Br J Nutr 2007; 97(3): 550-60.
[http://dx.doi.org/ 10.1017/S0007114507381324] [PMID: 17313718]

[182] Smedman A, Vessby B. Conjugated linoleic acid supplementation in humans--metabolic effects. Lipids 2001; 36(8): 773-81.
[http://dx.doi.org/ 10.1007/s11745-001-0784-7] [PMID: 11592727]

[183] Seidner DL, Lashner BA, Brzezinski A, *et al*. An oral supplement enriched with fish oil, soluble fiber, and antioxidants for corticosteroid sparing in ulcerative colitis: a randomized, controlled trial. Clin Gastroenterol Hepatol 2005; 3(4): 358-69.
[http://dx.doi.org/ 10.1016/S1542-3565(04)00672-X] [PMID: 15822041]

[184] Hsiao EY, McBride SW, Hsien S, *et al*. Microbiota modulate behavioral and physiological abnormalities associated with neurodevelopmental disorders. Cell 2013; 155(7): 1451-63.
[http://dx.doi.org/ 10.1016/j.cell.2013.11.024] [PMID: 24315484]

[185] Sridharan GV, Choi K, Klemashevich C, *et al*. Prediction and quantification of bioactive microbiota metabolites in the mouse gut. Nat Commun 2014; 5(1): 5492.
[http://dx.doi.org/ 10.1038/ncomms6492] [PMID: 25411059]

[186] Devlin AS, Marcobal A, Dodd D, *et al*. Modulation of a circulating uremic solute *via* rational genetic manipulation of the gut microbiota. Cell Host Microbe 2016; 20(6): 709-15.
[http://dx.doi.org/ 10.1016/j.chom.2016.10.021] [PMID: 27916477]

[187] Rothhammer V, Quintana FJ. The aryl hydrocarbon receptor: an environmental sensor integrating immune responses in health and disease. Nat Rev Immunol 2019; 19(3): 184-97.
[http://dx.doi.org/ 10.1038/s41577-019-0125-8] [PMID: 30718831]

[188] Metidji A, *et al*. The environmental sensor AHR protects from inflammatory damage by maintaining intestinal stem cell homeostasis and barrier integrity. 2018.
[http://dx.doi.org/ 10.1016/j.immuni.2018.07.010]

[189] Cervantes-Barragan L, Chai JN, Tianero MD, *et al*. *Lactobacillus reuteri* induces gut intraepithelial CD4⁻CD8αα⁺ T cells. Science 2017; 357(6353): 806-10.
[http://dx.doi.org/ 10.1126/science.aah5825] [PMID: 28775213]

[190] Zelante T, Iannitti RG, Cunha C, *et al*. Tryptophan catabolites from microbiota engage aryl hydrocarbon receptor and balance mucosal reactivity *via* interleukin-22. Immunity 2013; 39(2): 372-85.
[http://dx.doi.org/ 10.1016/j.immuni.2013.08.003] [PMID: 23973224]

[191] Beaumont M, Neyrinck AM, Olivares M, *et al*. The gut microbiota metabolite indole alleviates liver inflammation in mice. FASEB J 2018; 32(12): fj201800544.
[http://dx.doi.org/ 10.1096/fj.201800544] [PMID: 29906245]

[192] Rothhammer V, Mascanfroni ID, Bunse L, *et al*. Type I interferons and microbial metabolites of tryptophan modulate astrocyte activity and central nervous system inflammation *via* the aryl hydrocarbon receptor. Nat Med 2016; 22(6): 586-97.
[http://dx.doi.org/ 10.1038/nm.4106] [PMID: 27158906]

[193] Rothhammer V, Borucki DM, Tjon EC, *et al*. Microglial control of astrocytes in response to microbial metabolites. Nature 2018; 557(7707): 724-8.
[http://dx.doi.org/ 10.1038/s41586-018-0119-x] [PMID: 29769726]

[194] Apetoh L, Quintana FJ, Pot C, *et al*. The aryl hydrocarbon receptor interacts with c-Maf to promote the differentiation of type 1 regulatory T cells induced by IL-27. Nat Immunol 2010; 11(9): 854-61.
[http://dx.doi.org/ 10.1038/ni.1912] [PMID: 20676095]

[195]   Duranton F, Cohen G, De Smet R, *et al.* Normal and pathologic concentrations of uremic toxins. J Am
        Soc Nephrol 2012; 23(7): 1258-70.
        [http://dx.doi.org/ 10.1681/ASN.2011121175] [PMID: 22626821]

[196]   Nakano T, Katsuki S, Chen M, *et al.* Uremic toxin indoxyl sulfate promotes proinflammatory
        macrophage activation *via* the interplay of OATP2B1 and Dll4-Notch signaling: potential mechanism
        for accelerated atherogenesis in chronic kidney disease. Circulation 2019; 139(1): 78-96.
        [http://dx.doi.org/ 10.1161/CIRCULATIONAHA.118.034588] [PMID: 30586693]

[197]   Hamer HM, De Preter V, Windey K, Verbeke K. Functional analysis of colonic bacterial metabolism:
        relevant to health? Am J Physiol Gastrointest Liver Physiol 2012; 302(1): G1-9.
        [http://dx.doi.org/ 10.1152/ajpgi.00048.2011] [PMID: 22016433]

[198]   Opdebeeck B, Maudsley S, Azmi A, *et al.* Indoxyl sulfate and p-cresyl sulfate promote vascular
        calcification and associate with glucose intolerance. J Am Soc Nephrol 2019; 30(5): 751-66.
        [http://dx.doi.org/ 10.1681/ASN.2018060609] [PMID: 30940651]

[199]   Meijers BK, Van Kerckhoven S, Verbeke K, *et al.* The uremic retention solute p-cresyl sulfate and
        markers of endothelial damage. Am J Kidney Dis 2009; 54(5): 891-901.
        [http://dx.doi.org/ 10.1053/j.ajkd.2009.04.022] [PMID: 19615803]

[200]   Patel M, Fowler D, Sizer J, Walton C. Faecal volatile biomarkers of Clostridium difficile infection.
        PLoS One 2019; 14(4): e0215256.
        [http://dx.doi.org/ 10.1371/journal.pone.0215256] [PMID: 30986230]

[201]   Bammens B, Evenepoel P, Keuleers H, Verbeke K, Vanrenterghem Y. Free serum concentrations of
        the protein-bound retention solute p-cresol predict mortality in hemodialysis patients. Kidney Int 2006;
        69(6): 1081-7.
        [http://dx.doi.org/ 10.1038/sj.ki.5000115] [PMID: 16421516]

[202]   Wan Y, Wang F, Yuan J, *et al.* Effects of dietary fat on gut microbiota and faecal metabolites, and
        their relationship with cardiometabolic risk factors: a 6-month randomised controlled-feeding trial. Gut
        2019; 68(8): 1417-29.
        [http://dx.doi.org/ 10.1136/gutjnl-2018-317609] [PMID: 30782617]

[203]   De Preter V, Falony G, Windey K, Hamer HM, De Vuyst L, Verbeke K. The prebiotic, oligofructose-
        enriched inulin modulates the faecal metabolite profile: an *in vitro* analysis. Mol Nutr Food Res 2010;
        54(12): 1791-801.
        [http://dx.doi.org/ 10.1002/mnfr.201000136] [PMID: 20568238]

[204]   Lecerf J-M, Dépeint F, Clerc E, *et al.* Xylo-oligosaccharide (XOS) in combination with inulin
        modulates both the intestinal environment and immune status in healthy subjects, while XOS alone
        only shows prebiotic properties. Br J Nutr 2012; 108(10): 1847-58.
        [http://dx.doi.org/ 10.1017/S0007114511007252] [PMID: 22264499]

[205]   Cloetens L, Broekaert WF, Delaedt Y, *et al.* Tolerance of arabinoxylan-oligosaccharides and their
        prebiotic activity in healthy subjects: a randomised, placebo-controlled cross-over study. Br J Nutr
        2010; 103(5): 703-13.
        [http://dx.doi.org/ 10.1017/S0007114509992248] [PMID: 20003568]

[206]   Wahlström A, Sayin SI, Marschall H-U, Bäckhed F. Intestinal crosstalk between bile acids and
        microbiota and its impact on host metabolism. Cell Metab 2016; 24(1): 41-50.
        [http://dx.doi.org/ 10.1016/j.cmet.2016.05.005] [PMID: 27320064]

[207]   Yao L, Seaton SC, Ndousse-Fetter S, *et al.* A selective gut bacterial bile salt hydrolase alters host
        metabolism. eLife 2018; 7: e37182.
        [http://dx.doi.org/ 10.7554/eLife.37182] [PMID: 30014852]

[208]   Levy M, Thaiss CA, Zeevi D, *et al.* Microbiota-modulated metabolites shape the intestinal
        microenvironment by regulating NLRP6 inflammasome signaling. Cell 2015; 163(6): 1428-43.
        [http://dx.doi.org/ 10.1016/j.cell.2015.10.048] [PMID: 26638072]

[209] Yazici C, Wolf PG, Kim H, *et al.* Race-dependent association of sulfidogenic bacteria with colorectal cancer. Gut 2017; 66(11): 1983-94.
[http://dx.doi.org/ 10.1136/gutjnl-2016-313321] [PMID: 28153960]

[210] Olson CA, Vuong HE, Yano JM, Liang QY, Nusbaum DJ, Hsiao EY. The gut microbiota mediates the anti-seizure effects of the ketogenic diet. Cell 2018; 173(7): 1728-4.
[http://dx.doi.org/ 10.1016/j.cell.2018.04.027]

[211] Steed AL, Christophi GP, Kaiko GE, *et al.* The microbial metabolite desaminotyrosine protects from influenza through type I interferon. Science 2017; 357(6350): 498-502.
[http://dx.doi.org/ 10.1126/science.aam5336] [PMID: 28774928]

[212] Koh A, *et al.* Microbially produced imidazole propionate impairs insulin signaling through mTORC1. 2018.
[http://dx.doi.org/ 10.1016/j.cell.2018.09.055]

[213] Madeo F, Eisenberg T, Pietrocola F, Kroemer G. Spermidine in health and disease. Science 2018; 359(6374): eaan2788.
[http://dx.doi.org/ 10.1126/science.aan2788] [PMID: 29371440]

[214] Weiss TS, Herfarth H, Obermeier F, *et al.* Intracellular polyamine levels of intestinal epithelial cells in inflammatory bowel disease. Inflamm Bowel Dis 2004; 10(5): 529-35.
[http://dx.doi.org/ 10.1097/00054725-200409000-00006] [PMID: 15472512]

[215] Levy M, Shapiro H, Thaiss CA, Elinav E. NLRP6: a multifaceted innate immune sensor. Trends Immunol 2017; 38(4): 248-60.
[http://dx.doi.org/ 10.1016/j.it.2017.01.001] [PMID: 28214100]

[216] Thaiss CA, *et al.* Microbiota diurnal rhythmicity programs host transcriptome oscillations. 2016.
[http://dx.doi.org/ 10.1016/j.cell.2016.11.003]

[217] Thaiss CA, Levy M, Elinav E. Chronobiomics: the biological clock as a new principle in host–microbial interactions. PLoS Pathog 2015; 11(10): e1005113.
[http://dx.doi.org/ 10.1371/journal.ppat.1005113] [PMID: 26448621]

[218] Zwighaft Z, Aviram R, Shalev M, *et al.* Circadian clock control by polyamine levels through a mechanism that declines with age. Cell Metab 2015; 22(5): 874-85.
[http://dx.doi.org/ 10.1016/j.cmet.2015.09.011] [PMID: 26456331]

[219] Grizotte-Lake M, *et al.* Commensals suppress intestinal epithelial cell retinoic acid synthesis to regulate interleukin-22 activity and prevent microbial dysbiosis. 2018.
[http://dx.doi.org/ 10.1016/j.immuni.2018.11.018]

[220] Clemente JC, Manasson J, Scher JU. The role of the gut microbiome in systemic inflammatory disease. 2018.
[http://dx.doi.org/ 10.1136/bmj.j5145]

[221] Wada Y, Hisamatsu T, Kamada N, Okamoto S, Hibi T. Retinoic acid contributes to the induction of IL-12-hypoproducing dendritic cells. Inflamm Bowel Dis 2009; 15(10): 1548-56.
[http://dx.doi.org/ 10.1002/ibd.20934] [PMID: 19340880]

[222] Feng F-E, Feng R, Wang M, *et al.* Oral all-trans retinoic acid plus danazol *versus* danazol as second-line treatment in adults with primary immune thrombocytopenia: a multicentre, randomised, open-label, phase 2 trial. Lancet Haematol 2017; 4(10): e487-96.
[http://dx.doi.org/ 10.1016/S2352-3026(17)30170-9] [PMID: 28917657]

[223] Nozaki Y, Tamaki C, Yamagata T, *et al.* All-trans-retinoic acid suppresses interferon-γ and tumor necrosis factor-α; a possible therapeutic agent for rheumatoid arthritis. Rheumatol Int 2006; 26(9): 810-7.
[http://dx.doi.org/ 10.1007/s00296-005-0076-1] [PMID: 16292516]

[224] Smith MA, Adamson PC, Balis FM, *et al.* Phase I and pharmacokinetic evaluation of all-trans-retinoic

acid in pediatric patients with cancer. J Clin Oncol 1992; 10(11): 1666-73.
[http://dx.doi.org/ 10.1200/JCO.1992.10.11.1666] [PMID: 1403049]

[225] Abdelhamid L, Luo XM. Retinoic acid, leaky gut, and autoimmune diseases. Nutrients 2018; 10(8): 1016.
[http://dx.doi.org/ 10.3390/nu10081016] [PMID: 30081517]

[226] Urdaneta V, Casadesús J. Interactions between bacteria and bile salts in the gastrointestinal and hepatobiliary tracts. Front Med (Lausanne) 2017; 4: 163.
[http://dx.doi.org/ 10.3389/fmed.2017.00163] [PMID: 29043249]

[227] Ridlon JM, Kang D-J, Hylemon PB. Bile salt biotransformations by human intestinal bacteria. J Lipid Res 2006; 47(2): 241-59.
[http://dx.doi.org/ 10.1194/jlr.R500013-JLR200] [PMID: 16299351]

[228] Sayin SI, Wahlström A, Felin J, *et al.* Gut microbiota regulates bile acid metabolism by reducing the levels of tauro-beta-muricholic acid, a naturally occurring FXR antagonist. Cell Metab 2013; 17(2): 225-35.
[http://dx.doi.org/ 10.1016/j.cmet.2013.01.003] [PMID: 23395169]

[229] Selwyn FP, Csanaky IL, Zhang Y, Klaassen CD. Importance of large intestine in regulating bile acids and glucagon-like peptide-1 in germ-free mice. Drug Metab Dispos 2015; 43(10): 1544-56.
[http://dx.doi.org/ 10.1124/dmd.115.065276] [PMID: 26199423]

[230] Worthmann A, *et al.* Cold-induced conversion of cholesterol to bile acids in mice shapes the gut microbiome and promotes adaptive thermogenesis. 2017.
[http://dx.doi.org/ 10.1038/nm.4357]

[231] Weingarden AR, Chen C, Zhang N, *et al.* Ursodeoxycholic Acid Inhibits Clostridium difficile Spore Germination and Vegetative Growth, and Prevents the Recurrence of Ileal Pouchitis Associated With the Infection. J Clin Gastroenterol 2016; 50(8): 624-30.
[http://dx.doi.org/ 10.1097/MCG.0000000000000427] [PMID: 26485102]

[232] Jain U, *et al.* Temporal Regulation of the Bacterial Metabolite Deoxycholate during Colonic Repair Is Critical for Crypt Regeneration. 2018.
[http://dx.doi.org/ 10.1016/j.chom.2018.07.019]

[233] Ma C, Han M, Heinrich B, *et al.* Gut microbiome-mediated bile acid metabolism regulates liver cancer *via* NKT cells. Science 2018; 360(6391): eaan5931.
[http://dx.doi.org/ 10.1126/science.aan5931] [PMID: 29798856]

[234] Bayerdörffer E, Mannes GA, Ochsenkühn T, Dirschedl P, Wiebecke B, Paumgartner G. Unconjugated secondary bile acids in the serum of patients with colorectal adenomas. Gut 1995; 36(2): 268-73.
[http://dx.doi.org/ 10.1136/gut.36.2.268] [PMID: 7883228]

[235] Yoshimoto S, Loo TM, Atarashi K, *et al.* Obesity-induced gut microbial metabolite promotes liver cancer through senescence secretome. Nature 2013; 499(7456): 97-101.
[http://dx.doi.org/ 10.1038/nature12347] [PMID: 23803760]

[236] Braune A, Blaut M. Bacterial species involved in the conversion of dietary flavonoids in the human gut. Gut Microbes 2016; 7(3): 216-34.
[http://dx.doi.org/ 10.1080/19490976.2016.1158395] [PMID: 26963713]

[237] Cassidy A, Minihane A-M. The role of metabolism (and the microbiome) in defining the clinical efficacy of dietary flavonoids. Am J Clin Nutr 2017; 105(1): 10-22.
[http://dx.doi.org/ 10.3945/ajcn.116.136051] [PMID: 27881391]

[238] Thaiss CA, Itav S, Rothschild D, *et al.* Persistent microbiome alterations modulate the rate of post-dieting weight regain. Nature 2016; 540(7634): 544-51.
[http://dx.doi.org/ 10.1038/nature20796] [PMID: 27906159]

[239] Rodríguez Vaquero MJ, Manca de Nadra MC. Growth parameter and viability modifications of Escherichia coli by phenolic compounds and Argentine wine extracts. Appl Biochem Biotechnol 2008;

151(2-3): 342-52.
[http://dx.doi.org/ 10.1007/s12010-008-8197-0] [PMID: 18594776]

[240] Liu C, Ma J, Sun J, *et al.* Flavonoid-rich extract of Paulownia fortunei flowers attenuates diet-induced hyperlipidemia, hepatic steatosis and insulin resistance in obesity mice by AMPK pathway. Nutrients 2017; 9(9): 959.
[http://dx.doi.org/ 10.3390/nu9090959] [PMID: 28867797]

[241] Thaiss CA, Shapiro H, Elinav E. Post-dieting weight gain: the role of persistent microbiome changes. 2017.

[242] Weng Z, Patel A B, Panagiotidou S, Theoharides T C. The novel flavone tetramethoxyluteolin is a potent inhibitor of human mast cells 2015.
[http://dx.doi.org/ 10.1016/j.jaci.2014.10.032]

[243] Wang J, Ho L, Zhao W, *et al.* Grape-derived polyphenolics prevent Abeta oligomerization and attenuate cognitive deterioration in a mouse model of Alzheimer's disease. J Neurosci 2008; 28(25): 6388-92.
[http://dx.doi.org/ 10.1523/JNEUROSCI.0364-08.2008] [PMID: 18562609]

[244] Cohen LJ, Kang HS, Chu J, *et al.* Functional metagenomic discovery of bacterial effectors in the human microbiome and isolation of commendamide, a GPCR G2A/132 agonist. Proc Natl Acad Sci USA 2015; 112(35): E4825-34.
[http://dx.doi.org/ 10.1073/pnas.1508737112] [PMID: 26283367]

[245] Cohen LJ, Esterhazy D, Kim SH, *et al.* Commensal bacteria make GPCR ligands that mimic human signalling molecules. Nature 2017; 549(7670): 48-53.
[http://dx.doi.org/ 10.1038/nature23874] [PMID: 28854168]

[246] Descamps HC, Herrmann B, Wiredu D, Thaiss CA. The path toward using microbial metabolites as therapies. EBioMedicine 2019; 44: 747-54.
[http://dx.doi.org/ 10.1016/j.ebiom.2019.05.063] [PMID: 31201140]

[247] Palma ML, Zamith-Miranda D, Martins FS, *et al.* Probiotic Saccharomyces cerevisiae strains as biotherapeutic tools: is there room for improvement? Appl Microbiol Biotechnol 2015; 99(16): 6563-70.
[http://dx.doi.org/ 10.1007/s00253-015-6776-x] [PMID: 26142388]

[248] Brader P, Stritzker J, Riedl CC, *et al.* Escherichia coli Nissle 1917 facilitates tumor detection by positron emission tomography and optical imaging. Clin Cancer Res 2008; 14(8): 2295-302.
[http://dx.doi.org/ 10.1158/1078-0432.CCR-07-4254] [PMID: 18369089]

[249] Walter J. Ecological role of lactobacilli in the gastrointestinal tract: implications for fundamental and biomedical research. Appl Environ Microbiol 2008; 74(16): 4985-96.
[http://dx.doi.org/ 10.1128/AEM.00753-08] [PMID: 18539818]

[250] Candela M, Perna F, Carnevali P, *et al.* Interaction of probiotic Lactobacillus and *Bifidobacterium* strains with human intestinal epithelial cells: adhesion properties, competition against enteropathogens and modulation of IL-8 production. Int J Food Microbiol 2008; 125(3): 286-92.
[http://dx.doi.org/ 10.1016/j.ijfoodmicro.2008.04.012] [PMID: 18524406]

[251] Yan F, Cao H, Cover TL, Whitehead R, Washington MK, Polk DB. Soluble proteins produced by probiotic bacteria regulate intestinal epithelial cell survival and growth. Gastroenterology 2007; 132(2): 562-75.
[http://dx.doi.org/ 10.1053/j.gastro.2006.11.022] [PMID: 17258729]

[252] Ewaschuk JB, Diaz H, Meddings L, *et al.* Secreted bioactive factors from *Bifidobacterium* infantis enhance epithelial cell barrier function. Am J Physiol Gastrointest Liver Physiol 2008; 295(5): G1025-34.
[http://dx.doi.org/ 10.1152/ajpgi.90227.2008] [PMID: 18787064]

[253] Moghadam MS, Foo HL, Leow TC, Rahim RA, Loh TC. Novel bacteriocinogenic *Lactobacillus*

plantarum strains and their differentiation by sequence analysis of 16 S rDNA, 16 S-23 S and 23 S-5 S intergenic spacer regions and randomly amplified polymorphic DNA analysis. Food Technol Biotechnol 2010; 48(4): 476-83.

[254] Foo H, Lim Y, Rusul G. Isolation of bacteriocin producing lactic acid bacteria from Malaysian fermented food, Tapai Proceeding of the 11th World Congress of Food Sciences and Technology. Seoul, Korea. 2001.

[255] Foo H, Loh T, Lai P, Lim Y, Kufli C, Rusul G. Effects of adding *Lactobacillus plantarum* I-UL4 metabolites in drinking water of rats. Pak J Nutr 2003; 2(5): 283-8.
[http://dx.doi.org/ 10.3923/pjn.2003.283.288]

[256] Loh T, Lee T, Foo H, Law F, Ajion M. Growth performance and fecal microflora of rats offered metabolites from lactic acid bacteria. J Appl Anim Res 2008; 34(1): 61-4.
[http://dx.doi.org/ 10.1080/09712119.2008.9706941]

[257] Tai HF, Foo HL, Abdul Rahim R, Loh TC, Abdullah MP, Yoshinobu K. Molecular characterisation of new organisation of plnEF and plw loci of bacteriocin genes harbour concomitantly in *Lactobacillus plantarum* I-UL4. Microb Cell Fact 2015; 14(1): 89.
[http://dx.doi.org/ 10.1186/s12934-015-0280-y] [PMID: 26077560]

[258] Cuevas-González PF, Liceaga AM, Aguilar-Toalá JE. Postbiotics and paraprobiotics: From concepts to applications. Food Res Int 2020; 136: 109502.
[http://dx.doi.org/ 10.1016/j.foodres.2020.109502] [PMID: 32846581]

[259] Raz E, Rachmilewitz D. Inactivated probiotic bacteria and methods of use thereof. 2005.

[260] Gould G. Heat-induced injury and inactivation. 1989.

[261] Juneja VK. Thermal inactivation of microorganisms. FOOD SCIENCE AND TECHNOLOGY-NEW YORK-MARCEL DEKKER 2002; pp. 13-54.

[262] Ivec M, Botić T, Koren S, Jakobsen M, Weingartl H, Cencič A. Interactions of macrophages with probiotic bacteria lead to increased antiviral response against vesicular stomatitis virus. Antiviral Res 2007; 75(3): 266-74.
[http://dx.doi.org/ 10.1016/j.antiviral.2007.03.013] [PMID: 17512614]

[263] József L, Khreiss T, Filep JG. CpG motifs in bacterial DNA delay apoptosis of neutrophil granulocytes. FASEB J 2004; 18(14): 1776-8.
[http://dx.doi.org/ 10.1096/fj.04-2048fje] [PMID: 15345690]

[264] Ou CC, Lin SL, Tsai JJ, Lin MY. Heat-killed lactic acid bacteria enhance immunomodulatory potential by skewing the immune response toward Th1 polarization. J Food Sci 2011; 76(5): M260-7.
[http://dx.doi.org/ 10.1111/j.1750-3841.2011.02161.x] [PMID: 22417436]

[265] Moradi M, Molaei R, Guimarães JT. A review on preparation and chemical analysis of postbiotics from lactic acid bacteria. Enzyme Microb Technol 2021; 143: 109722.
[http://dx.doi.org/ 10.1016/j.enzmictec.2020.109722] [PMID: 33375981]

[266] Kawase M, He F, Kubota A, Yoda K, Miyazawa K, Hiramatsu M. Heat-killed *Lactobacillus gasseri* TMC0356 protects mice against influenza virus infection by stimulating gut and respiratory immune responses. FEMS Immunol Med Microbiol 2012; 64(2): 280-8.
[http://dx.doi.org/ 10.1111/j.1574-695X.2011.00903.x] [PMID: 22098223]

[267] Dash G, Raman RP, Pani Prasad K, Makesh M, Pradeep MA, Sen S. Evaluation of paraprobiotic applicability of *Lactobacillus plantarum* in improving the immune response and disease protection in giant freshwater prawn, Macrobrachium rosenbergii (de Man, 1879). Fish Shellfish Immunol 2015; 43(1): 167-74.
[http://dx.doi.org/ 10.1016/j.fsi.2014.12.007] [PMID: 25542379]

[268] Román L, Real F, Sorroza L, *et al.* The *in vitro* effect of probiotic Vagococcus fluvialis on the innate immune parameters of Sparus aurata and Dicentrarchus labrax. Fish Shellfish Immunol 2012; 33(5): 1071-5.

[http://dx.doi.org/ 10.1016/j.fsi.2012.06.028] [PMID: 22864109]

[269] Kamilya D, Baruah A, Sangma T, Chowdhury S, Pal P. Inactivated probiotic bacteria stimulate cellular immune responses of catla, Catla catla (Hamilton) *in vitro*. Probiotics Antimicrob Proteins 2015; 7(2): 101-6.
[http://dx.doi.org/ 10.1007/s12602-015-9191-9] [PMID: 25736432]

[270] Zheng X, Duan Y, Dong H, Zhang J. Effects of dietary *Lactobacillus plantarum* in different treatments on growth performance and immune gene expression of white shrimp Litopenaeus vannamei under normal condition and stress of acute low salinity. Fish Shellfish Immunol 2017; 62: 195-201.
[http://dx.doi.org/ 10.1016/j.fsi.2017.01.015] [PMID: 28108342]

[271] Panigrahi A, Viswanath K, Satoh S. Real time quantification of the immune gene expression in rainbow trout fed different forms of probiotic bacteria *Lactobacillus rhamnosus*. Aquacult Res 2011; 42(7): 906-17.
[http://dx.doi.org/ 10.1111/j.1365-2109.2010.02633.x]

[272] Muñoz-Atienza E, Araújo C, Lluch N, *et al.* Different impact of heat-inactivated and viable lactic acid bacteria of aquatic origin on turbot (*Scophthalmus maximus* L.) head-kidney leucocytes. Fish Shellfish Immunol 2015; 44(1): 214-23.
[http://dx.doi.org/ 10.1016/j.fsi.2015.02.021] [PMID: 25707601]

[273] Giri SS, Sen SS, Jun JW, Park SC, Sukumaran V. Heat-killed whole-cell products of the probiotic Pseudomonas aeruginosa VSG2 strain affect *in vitro* cytokine expression in head kidney macrophages of Labeo rohita. Fish Shellfish Immunol 2016; 50: 310-6.
[http://dx.doi.org/ 10.1016/j.fsi.2016.02.007] [PMID: 26876356]

[274] Yan YY, Xia HQ, Yang HL, Hoseinifar S, Sun YZ. Effects of dietary live or heat inactivated autochthonous Bacillus pumilus SE 5 on growth performance, immune responses and immune gene expression in grouper *Epinephelus coioides*. Aquacult Nutr 2016; 22(3): 698-707.
[http://dx.doi.org/ 10.1111/anu.12297]

[275] Biswas G, Korenaga H, Nagamine R, *et al.* Cytokine responses in the Japanese pufferfish (Takifugu rubripes) head kidney cells induced with heat-killed probiotics isolated from the Mongolian dairy products. Fish Shellfish Immunol 2013; 34(5): 1170-7.
[http://dx.doi.org/ 10.1016/j.fsi.2013.01.024] [PMID: 23422813]

[276] Biswas G, Korenaga H, Nagamine R, *et al.* Cytokine mediated immune responses in the Japanese pufferfish (Takifugu rubripes) administered with heat-killed *Lactobacillus paracasei* spp. paracasei (06TCa22) isolated from the Mongolian dairy product. Int Immunopharmacol 2013; 17(2): 358-65.
[http://dx.doi.org/ 10.1016/j.intimp.2013.06.030] [PMID: 23867289]

[277] Pan X, Wu T, Song Z, Tang H, Zhao Z. Immune responses and enhanced disease resistance in Chinese drum, Miichthys miiuy (Basilewsky), after oral administration of live or dead cells of Clostridium butyrium CB2. J Fish Dis 2008; 31(9): 679-86.
[http://dx.doi.org/ 10.1111/j.1365-2761.2008.00955.x] [PMID: 18786030]

[278] Mukhopadhyay S, Ramaswamy R. Application of emerging technologies to control Salmonella in foods: A review. Food Res Int 2012; 45(2): 666-77.
[http://dx.doi.org/ 10.1016/j.foodres.2011.05.016]

[279] Gayán E, Álvarez I, Condón S. Inactivation of bacterial spores by UV-C light. Innov Food Sci Emerg Technol 2013; 19: 140-5.
[http://dx.doi.org/ 10.1016/j.ifset.2013.04.007]

[280] Franz CM, Specht I, Cho G-S, Graef V, Stahl MR. UV-C-inactivation of microorganisms in naturally cloudy apple juice using novel inactivation equipment based on Dean vortex technology. Food Control 2009; 20(12): 1103-7.
[http://dx.doi.org/ 10.1016/j.foodcont.2009.02.010]

[281] Román L, Real F, Padilla D, *et al.* Cytokine expression in head-kidney leucocytes of European sea bass (Dicentrarchus labrax L.) after incubation with the probiotic Vagococcus fluvialis L-21. Fish

Shellfish Immunol 2013; 35(4): 1329-32.
[http://dx.doi.org/ 10.1016/j.fsi.2013.07.036] [PMID: 23927874]

[282] Rad AH, Abbasi A, Kafil HS, Ganbarov K. Potential Pharmaceutical and Food Applications of Postbiotics: A Review. Curr Pharm Biotechnol 2020; 21(15): 1576-87.
[http://dx.doi.org/ 10.2174/1389201021666200516154833] [PMID: 32416671]

[283] Favero M. Chemical disinfection of medical and surgical materials. 1991.

[284] Choudhury TG, Kamilya D. Paraprobiotics: an aquaculture perspective. Rev Aquacult 2019; 11(4): 1258-70.
[http://dx.doi.org/ 10.1111/raq.12290]

[285] Niamah A K. Ultrasound treatment (low frequency) effects on probiotic bacteria growth in fermented milk 2019.

[286] Butz P, Tauscher B. Emerging technologies: chemical aspects. Food Res Int 2002; 35(2-3): 279-84.
[http://dx.doi.org/ 10.1016/S0963-9969(01)00197-1]

[287] da Cruz Cabral L, Fernández Pinto V, Patriarca A. Application of plant derived compounds to control fungal spoilage and mycotoxin production in foods. Int J Food Microbiol 2013; 166(1): 1-14.
[http://dx.doi.org/ 10.1016/j.ijfoodmicro.2013.05.026] [PMID: 23816820]

[288] Ross AI, Griffiths MW, Mittal GS, Deeth HC. Combining nonthermal technologies to control foodborne microorganisms. Int J Food Microbiol 2003; 89(2-3): 125-38.
[http://dx.doi.org/ 10.1016/S0168-1605(03)00161-2] [PMID: 14623378]

[289] Dinić M, Lukić J, Djokić J, *et al.* Lactobacillus fermentum postbiotic-induced autophagy as potential approach for treatment of acetaminophen hepatotoxicity. Front Microbiol 2017; 8: 594.
[http://dx.doi.org/ 10.3389/fmicb.2017.00594] [PMID: 28428777]

[290] Ma EL, Choi YJ, Choi J, Pothoulakis C, Rhee SH, Im E. The anticancer effect of probiotic Bacillus polyfermenticus on human colon cancer cells is mediated through ErbB2 and ErbB3 inhibition. Int J Cancer 2010; 127(4): 780-90.
[PMID: 19876926]

[291] Ooi MF, *et al.* Effects of carbon and nitrogen sources on bacteriocin-inhibitory activity of postbiotic metabolites produced by *Lactobacillus plantarum* I-UL4. Malays J Microbiol 2015; 11(2): 176-84.

[292] Tan HK, Foo HL, Loh TC, Alitheen NBM, Rahim RA. Cytotoxic effect of proteinaceous postbiotic metabolites produced by *Lactobacillus plantarum* I-UL4 cultivated in different media composition on MCF-7 breast cancer cell. Malays J Microbiol 2015; 11(2): 207-14.

[293] Foo H, Loh T, Law F, Lim Y, Kufli C, Rusul G. Effects of feeding *Lactobacillus plantarum* I-UL4 isolated from Malaysian Tempeh on growth performance, faecal flora and lactic acid bacteria and plasma cholesterol concentrations in postweaning rats. Food Sci Biotechnol 2003; 12(4): 403-8.

[294] De Vuyst L, Leroy F. Bacteriocins from lactic acid bacteria: production, purification, and food applications. J Mol Microbiol Biotechnol 2007; 13(4): 194-9.
[http://dx.doi.org/ 10.1159/000104752] [PMID: 17827969]

[295] Saraniya A, Jeevaratnam K. Optimization of nutritional and non--nutritional factors involved for production of antimicrobial compounds from *Lactobacillus pentosus* SJ65 using response surface methodology. Braz J Microbiol 2014; 45(1): 81-8.
[http://dx.doi.org/ 10.1590/S1517-83822014000100012] [PMID: 24948917]

[296] Malheiros PS, Sant'Anna V, Todorov SD, Franco BD. Optimization of growth and bacteriocin production by Lactobacillus sakei subsp. sakei2a. Braz J Microbiol 2015; 46(3): 825-34.
[PMID: 26413066]

[297] Li J-Y, Zhang LW, Du M, *et al.* Effect of tween series on growth and Cis-9, trans-11 conjugated linoleic acid production of *Lactobacillus acidophilus* F0221 in the presence of bile salts. Int J Mol Sci 2011; 12(12): 9138-54.

[http://dx.doi.org/ 10.3390/ijms12129138] [PMID: 22272124]

[298] S Hayek, S Ibrahim. Current limitations and challenges with lactic acid bacteria: A review. Food Nutr Sci 2013; 4(11): 73-87.
[http://dx.doi.org/ 10.4236/fns.2013.411A010]

[299] Pyclik M, Srutkova D, Schwarzer M, Górska S. Bifidobacteria cell wall-derived exo-polysaccharides, lipoteichoic acids, peptidoglycans, polar lipids and proteins - their chemical structure and biological attributes. Int J Biol Macromol 2020; 147: 333-49.
[http://dx.doi.org/ 10.1016/j.ijbiomac.2019.12.227] [PMID: 31899242]

[300] Saadat Y R, Gargari B P, Shahabi A, Nami Y, Khosroushahi A Y. Prophylactic role of Lactobacillus paracasei exopolysaccharides on colon cancer cells through apoptosis not ferroptosis 2020.

[301] Schumann P. Peptidoglycan structure 2011.
[http://dx.doi.org/ 10.1016/B978-0-12-387730-7.00005-X]

[302] Veerkamp JH. The structure of the cell wall peptidoglycan of *Bifidobacterium* bifidum var. pennsylvanicus. Arch Biochem Biophys 1971; 143(1): 204-11.
[http://dx.doi.org/ 10.1016/0003-9861(71)90200-1] [PMID: 4254496]

[303] Kok MG, Ruijken MM, Swann JR, Wilson ID, Somsen GW, de Jong GJ. Anionic metabolic profiling of urine from antibiotic-treated rats by capillary electrophoresis-mass spectrometry. Anal Bioanal Chem 2013; 405(8): 2585-94.
[http://dx.doi.org/ 10.1007/s00216-012-6701-4] [PMID: 23314487]

[304] Antunes LCM, Han J, Ferreira RB, Lolić P, Borchers CH, Finlay BB. Effect of antibiotic treatment on the intestinal metabolome. Antimicrob Agents Chemother 2011; 55(4): 1494-503.
[http://dx.doi.org/ 10.1128/AAC.01664-10] [PMID: 21282433]

[305] Want EJ, Cravatt BF, Siuzdak G. The expanding role of mass spectrometry in metabolite profiling and characterization. ChemBioChem 2005; 6(11): 1941-51.
[http://dx.doi.org/ 10.1002/cbic.200500151] [PMID: 16206229]

[306] Xiao JF, Zhou B, Ressom HW. Metabolite identification and quantitation in LC-MS/MS-based metabolomics. Trends Analyt Chem 2012; 32: 1-14.
[http://dx.doi.org/ 10.1016/j.trac.2011.08.009] [PMID: 22345829]

[307] Erickson AR, Cantarel BL, Lamendella R, *et al.* Integrated metagenomics/metaproteomics reveals human host-microbiota signatures of Crohn's disease. PLoS One 2012; 7(11): e49138.
[http://dx.doi.org/ 10.1371/journal.pone.0049138] [PMID: 23209564]

[308] Väremo L, Nookaew I, Nielsen J. Novel insights into obesity and diabetes through genome-scale metabolic modeling. Front Physiol 2013; 4: 92.
[http://dx.doi.org/ 10.3389/fphys.2013.00092] [PMID: 23630502]

[309] Sigurdsson MI, Jamshidi N, Steingrimsson E, Thiele I, Palsson BØ. A detailed genome-wide reconstruction of mouse metabolism based on human Recon 1. BMC Syst Biol 2010; 4(1): 140.
[http://dx.doi.org/ 10.1186/1752-0509-4-140] [PMID: 20959003]

[310] Karlsson FH, Nookaew I, Petranovic D, Nielsen J. Prospects for systems biology and modeling of the gut microbiome. 2011.
[http://dx.doi.org/ 10.1016/j.tibtech.2011.01.009]

[311] Borenstein E. Computational systems biology and in silico modeling of the human microbiome. Brief Bioinform 2012; 13(6): 769-80.
[http://dx.doi.org/ 10.1093/bib/bbs022] [PMID: 22589385]

[312] Chen N, del Val IJ, Kyriakopoulos S, Polizzi KM, Kontoravdi C. Metabolic network reconstruction: advances in in silico interpretation of analytical information. Curr Opin Biotechnol 2012; 23(1): 77-82.
[http://dx.doi.org/ 10.1016/j.copbio.2011.10.015] [PMID: 22119273]

[313] Greenblum S, Turnbaugh PJ, Borenstein E. Metagenomic systems biology of the human gut

microbiome reveals topological shifts associated with obesity and inflammatory bowel disease. Proc Natl Acad Sci USA 2012; 109(2): 594-9.
[http://dx.doi.org/ 10.1073/pnas.1116053109] [PMID: 22184244]

[314] Van Duynhoven J, *et al.* Metabolic fate of polyphenols in the human superorganism Proceedings of the national academy of sciences. vol. 108: 4531-8.
[http://dx.doi.org/ 10.1073/pnas.1000098107]

[315] Heinken A, Sahoo S, Fleming RM, Thiele I. Systems-level characterization of a host-microbe metabolic symbiosis in the mammalian gut. Gut Microbes 2013; 4(1): 28-40.
[http://dx.doi.org/ 10.4161/gmic.22370] [PMID: 23022739]

[316] Moriya Y, *et al.* PathPred: an enzyme-catalyzed metabolic pathway prediction server 2010.
[http://dx.doi.org/ 10.1093/nar/gkq318]

[317] Yousofshahi M, Lee K, Hassoun S. Probabilistic pathway construction. Metab Eng 2011; 13(4): 435-44.
[http://dx.doi.org/ 10.1016/j.ymben.2011.01.006] [PMID: 21292021]

[318] Ibrahim M, Anishetty S. A meta-metabolome network of carbohydrate metabolism: interactions between gut microbiota and host. Biochem Biophys Res Commun 2012; 428(2): 278-84.
[http://dx.doi.org/ 10.1016/j.bbrc.2012.10.045] [PMID: 23085046]

[319] Consortium HMP. Structure, function and diversity of the healthy human microbiome. Nature 2012; 486(7402): 207-14.
[http://dx.doi.org/ 10.1038/nature11234] [PMID: 22699609]

[320] Lynch SV, Pedersen O. The human intestinal microbiome in health and disease. N Engl J Med 2016; 375(24): 2369-79.
[http://dx.doi.org/ 10.1056/NEJMra1600266] [PMID: 27974040]

[321] Quraishi MN, Widlak M, Bhala N, *et al.* Systematic review with meta-analysis: the efficacy of faecal microbiota transplantation for the treatment of recurrent and refractory Clostridium difficile infection. Aliment Pharmacol Ther 2017; 46(5): 479-93.
[http://dx.doi.org/ 10.1111/apt.14201] [PMID: 28707337]

[322] Franzosa E A, *et al.* Gut microbiome structure and metabolic activity in inflammatory bowel disease 2019.
[http://dx.doi.org/ 10.1038/s41564-018-0306-4]

[323] Skelly AN, Sato Y, Kearney S, Honda K. Mining the microbiota for microbial and metabolite-based immunotherapies. Nat Rev Immunol 2019; 19(5): 305-23.
[http://dx.doi.org/ 10.1038/s41577-019-0144-5] [PMID: 30858494]

[324] Blacher E, Levy M, Tatirovsky E, Elinav E. Microbiome-modulated metabolites at the interface of host immunity. J Immunol 2017; 198(2): 572-80.
[http://dx.doi.org/ 10.4049/jimmunol.1601247] [PMID: 28069752]

[325] Michallet M-C, Rota G, Maslowski K, Guarda G. Innate receptors for adaptive immunity. Curr Opin Microbiol 2013; 16(3): 296-302.
[http://dx.doi.org/ 10.1016/j.mib.2013.04.003] [PMID: 23659869]

[326] Scheppach W. Treatment of distal ulcerative colitis with short-chain fatty acid enemas. A placebo-controlled trial. Dig Dis Sci 1996; 41(11): 2254-9.
[http://dx.doi.org/ 10.1007/BF02071409] [PMID: 8943981]

[327] Butzner JD, Parmar R, Bell CJ, Dalal V. Butyrate enema therapy stimulates mucosal repair in experimental colitis in the rat. Gut 1996; 38(4): 568-73.
[http://dx.doi.org/ 10.1136/gut.38.4.568] [PMID: 8707089]

[328] Macia L, Tan J, Vieira AT, *et al.* Metabolite-sensing receptors GPR43 and GPR109A facilitate dietary fibre-induced gut homeostasis through regulation of the inflammasome. Nat Commun 2015; 6: 6734.
[http://dx.doi.org/ 10.1038/ncomms7734] [PMID: 25828455]

[329] Plovier H, Cani PD. Enteroendocrine cells: metabolic relays between microbes and their host. Developmental Biology of Gastrointestinal Hormones. Karger Publishers 2017; Vol. 32: pp. 139-64.
[http://dx.doi.org/ 10.1159/000475736]

[330] Levy M, Blacher E, Elinav E. Microbiome, metabolites and host immunity. Curr Opin Microbiol 2017; 35: 8-15.
[http://dx.doi.org/ 10.1016/j.mib.2016.10.003] [PMID: 27883933]

[331] Morrison DJ, Preston T. Formation of short chain fatty acids by the gut microbiota and their impact on human metabolism. Gut Microbes 2016; 7(3): 189-200.
[http://dx.doi.org/ 10.1080/19490976.2015.1134082] [PMID: 26963409]

[332] Zheng X, Xie G, Zhao A, *et al.* The footprints of gut microbial-mammalian co-metabolism. J Proteome Res 2011; 10(12): 5512-22.
[http://dx.doi.org/ 10.1021/pr2007945] [PMID: 21970572]

[333] Robles-Vera I, Toral M, Romero M, *et al.* Antihypertensive effects of probiotics. Curr Hypertens Rep 2017; 19(4): 26.
[http://dx.doi.org/ 10.1007/s11906-017-0723-4] [PMID: 28315049]

[334] Konstantinov SR, Kuipers EJ, Peppelenbosch MP. Functional genomic analyses of the gut microbiota for CRC screening. Nat Rev Gastroenterol Hepatol 2013; 10(12): 741-5.
[http://dx.doi.org/ 10.1038/nrgastro.2013.178] [PMID: 24042452]

[335] Tsilingiri K, Rescigno M. Postbiotics: what else? Benef Microbes 2013; 4(1): 101-7.
[http://dx.doi.org/ 10.3920/BM2012.0046] [PMID: 23271068]

[336] Klemashevich C, Wu C, Howsmon D, Alaniz RC, Lee K, Jayaraman A. Rational identification of diet-derived postbiotics for improving intestinal microbiota function. Curr Opin Biotechnol 2014; 26: 85-90.
[http://dx.doi.org/ 10.1016/j.copbio.2013.10.006] [PMID: 24679263]

[337] Compare D, Rocco A, Coccoli P, *et al. Lactobacillus casei* DG and its postbiotic reduce the inflammatory mucosal response: an *ex-vivo* organ culture model of post-infectious irritable bowel syndrome. BMC Gastroenterol 2017; 17(1): 53.
[http://dx.doi.org/ 10.1186/s12876-017-0605-x] [PMID: 28410580]

[338] Haileselassie Y, Navis M, Vu N, Qazi KR, Rethi B, Sverremark-Ekström E. Postbiotic modulation of retinoic acid imprinted mucosal-like dendritic cells by probiotic *Lactobacillus reuteri* 17938 *in vitro.* Front Immunol 2016; 7: 96.
[http://dx.doi.org/ 10.3389/fimmu.2016.00096] [PMID: 27014275]

[339] Sokol H, Pigneur B, Watterlot L, *et al.* Faecalibacterium prausnitzii is an anti-inflammatory commensal bacterium identified by gut microbiota analysis of Crohn disease patients. Proc Natl Acad Sci USA 2008; 105(43): 16731-6.
[http://dx.doi.org/ 10.1073/pnas.0804812105] [PMID: 18936492]

[340] Tsilingiri K, Barbosa T, Penna G, *et al.* Probiotic and postbiotic activity in health and disease: comparison on a novel polarised *ex-vivo* organ culture model. Gut 2012; 61(7): 1007-15.
[http://dx.doi.org/ 10.1136/gutjnl-2011-300971] [PMID: 22301383]

[341] Cicenia A, Santangelo F, Gambardella L, *et al.* Protective role of postbiotic mediators secreted by *Lactobacillus rhamnosus* GG *versus* lipopolysaccharide-induced damage in human colonic smooth muscle cells. J Clin Gastroenterol 2016; 50 (Suppl 2, Proceedings from the 8th Probiotics, Prebiotics & New Foods for Microbiota and Human Health meeting held in Rome, Italy on September 13-15, 2015): S140-4.
[http://dx.doi.org/ 10.1097/MCG.0000000000000681] [PMID: 27741159]

[342] Kareem KY, Hooi Ling F, Teck Chwen L, May Foong O, Anjas Asmara S. Inhibitory activity of postbiotic produced by strains of *Lactobacillus plantarum* using reconstituted media supplemented with inulin. Gut Pathog 2014; 6(1): 23.

[http://dx.doi.org/ 10.1186/1757-4749-6-23] [PMID: 24991236]

[343] Xu R, Shang N, Li P. In vitro and *in vivo* antioxidant activity of exopolysaccharide fractions from *Bifidobacterium* animalis RH. Anaerobe 2011; 17(5): 226-31.
[http://dx.doi.org/ 10.1016/j.anaerobe.2011.07.010] [PMID: 21875680]

[344] Li W, Ji J, Chen X, Jiang M, Rui X, Dong M. Structural elucidation and antioxidant activities of exopolysaccharides from *Lactobacillus helveticus* MB2-1. Carbohydr Polym 2014; 102: 351-9.
[http://dx.doi.org/ 10.1016/j.carbpol.2013.11.053] [PMID: 24507291]

[345] Kim H, *et al. In vitro* antioxidative properties of lactobacilli. Asian-Australas J Anim Sci 2005; 19(2): 262-5.
[http://dx.doi.org/ 10.5713/ajas.2006.262]

[346] Li S, Zhao Y, Zhang L, *et al.* Antioxidant activity of *Lactobacillus plantarum* strains isolated from traditional Chinese fermented foods. Food Chem 2012; 135(3): 1914-9.
[http://dx.doi.org/ 10.1016/j.foodchem.2012.06.048] [PMID: 22953940]

[347] Lebeer S, Claes IJ, Vanderleyden J. Anti-inflammatory potential of probiotics: lipoteichoic acid makes a difference. Trends Microbiol 2012; 20(1): 5-10.
[http://dx.doi.org/ 10.1016/j.tim.2011.09.004] [PMID: 22030243]

[348] Yi Z-J, Fu Y-R, Li M, Gao K-S, Zhang X-G. Effect of LTA isolated from bifidobacteria on D-galactose-induced aging. Exp Gerontol 2009; 44(12): 760-5.
[http://dx.doi.org/ 10.1016/j.exger.2009.08.011] [PMID: 19735715]

[349] Oberg TS, Ward RE, Steele JL, Broadbent JR. Identification of plasmalogens in the cytoplasmic membrane of *Bifidobacterium* animalis subsp. lactis. Appl Environ Microbiol 2012; 78(3): 880-4.
[http://dx.doi.org/ 10.1128/AEM.06968-11] [PMID: 22138986]

[350] Oberg TS, Steele JL, Ingham SC, *et al.* Intrinsic and inducible resistance to hydrogen peroxide in *Bifidobacterium* species. J Ind Microbiol Biotechnol 2011; 38(12): 1947-53.
[http://dx.doi.org/ 10.1007/s10295-011-0983-y] [PMID: 21626209]

[351] Canfora EE, Jocken JW, Blaak EE. Short-chain fatty acids in control of body weight and insulin sensitivity. Nat Rev Endocrinol 2015; 11(10): 577-91.
[http://dx.doi.org/ 10.1038/nrendo.2015.128] [PMID: 26260141]

[352] Kimura I, Ozawa K, Inoue D, *et al.* The gut microbiota suppresses insulin-mediated fat accumulation *via* the short-chain fatty acid receptor GPR43. Nat Commun 2013; 4(1): 1829.
[http://dx.doi.org/ 10.1038/ncomms2852] [PMID: 23652017]

[353] den Besten G, van Eunen K, Groen AK, Venema K, Reijngoud D-J, Bakker BM. The role of short-chain fatty acids in the interplay between diet, gut microbiota, and host energy metabolism. J Lipid Res 2013; 54(9): 2325-40.
[http://dx.doi.org/ 10.1194/jlr.R036012] [PMID: 23821742]

[354] Sharma S, Singh RL, Kakkar P. Modulation of Bax/Bcl-2 and caspases by probiotics during acetaminophen induced apoptosis in primary hepatocytes. Food Chem Toxicol 2011; 49(4): 770-9.
[http://dx.doi.org/ 10.1016/j.fct.2010.11.041] [PMID: 21130831]

[355] Canonici A, Siret C, Pellegrino E, *et al.* Saccharomyces boulardii improves intestinal cell restitution through activation of the α2β1 integrin collagen receptor. PLoS One 2011; 6(3): e18427.
[http://dx.doi.org/ 10.1371/journal.pone.0018427] [PMID: 21483797]

[356] Thanh NT, Chwen LT, Foo HL, Hair-Bejo M, Kasim AB. Inhibitory activity of metabolites produced by strains of *Lactobacillus plantarum* isolated from Malaysian fermented food. Int J Probiotics Prebiotics 2010; 5(1): 37.

[357] Ogawa A, Kadooka Y, Kato K, Shirouchi B, Sato M. *Lactobacillus gasseri* SBT2055 reduces postprandial and fasting serum non-esterified fatty acid levels in Japanese hypertriacylglycerolemic subjects. Lipids Health Dis 2014; 13(1): 36.
[http://dx.doi.org/ 10.1186/1476-511X-13-36] [PMID: 24548293]

[358] Nakamura F, Ishida Y, Sawada D, *et al.* Fragmented lactic Acid bacterial cells activate peroxisome proliferator-activated receptors and ameliorate Dyslipidemia in obese mice. J Agric Food Chem 2016; 64(12): 2549-59.
[http://dx.doi.org/ 10.1021/acs.jafc.5b05827] [PMID: 26927959]

[359] Chi W, Dao D, Lau TC, *et al.* Bacterial peptidoglycan stimulates adipocyte lipolysis *via* NOD1. PLoS One 2014; 9(5): e97675.
[http://dx.doi.org/ 10.1371/journal.pone.0097675] [PMID: 24828250]

[360] Saadat YR, Khosroushahi AY, Movassaghpour AA, Talebi M, Gargari BP. Modulatory role of exopolysaccharides of Kluyveromyces marxianus and Pichia kudriavzevii as probiotic yeasts from dairy products in human colon cancer cells. J Funct Foods 2020; 64: 103675.
[http://dx.doi.org/ 10.1016/j.jff.2019.103675]

[361] Escamilla J, Lane MA, Maitin V. Cell-free supernatants from probiotic Lactobacillus casei and *Lactobacillus rhamnosus* GG decrease colon cancer cell invasion *in vitro.* Nutr Cancer 2012; 64(6): 871-8.
[http://dx.doi.org/ 10.1080/01635581.2012.700758] [PMID: 22830611]

[362] Kullisaar T, Zilmer M, Mikelsaar M, *et al.* Two antioxidative lactobacilli strains as promising probiotics. Int J Food Microbiol 2002; 72(3): 215-24.
[http://dx.doi.org/ 10.1016/S0168-1605(01)00674-2] [PMID: 11845820]

[363] Lin M-Y, Chang F-J. Antioxidative effect of intestinal bacteria *Bifidobacterium longum* ATCC 15708 and *Lactobacillus acidophilus* ATCC 4356. Dig Dis Sci 2000; 45(8): 1617-22.
[http://dx.doi.org/ 10.1023/A:1005577330695] [PMID: 11007114]

[364] Saide JA, Gilliland SE. Antioxidative activity of lactobacilli measured by oxygen radical absorbance capacity. J Dairy Sci 2005; 88(4): 1352-7.
[http://dx.doi.org/ 10.3168/jds.S0022-0302(05)72801-0] [PMID: 15778302]

[365] Shimamura S, Abe F, Ishibashi N, *et al.* Relationship between oxygen sensitivity and oxygen metabolism of *Bifidobacterium* species. J Dairy Sci 1992; 75(12): 3296-306.
[http://dx.doi.org/ 10.3168/jds.S0022-0302(92)78105-3] [PMID: 1474198]

[366] Yoon YH, Byun JR. Occurrence of glutathione sulphydryl (GSH) and antioxidant activities in probiotic Lactobacillus spp. Asian-Australas J Anim Sci 2004; 17(11): 1582-5.
[http://dx.doi.org/ 10.5713/ajas.2004.1582]

[367] Amaretti A, di Nunzio M, Pompei A, Raimondi S, Rossi M, Bordoni A. Antioxidant properties of potentially probiotic bacteria: *in vitro* and *in vivo* activities. Appl Microbiol Biotechnol 2013; 97(2): 809-17.
[http://dx.doi.org/ 10.1007/s00253-012-4241-7] [PMID: 22790540]

[368] Pan D, Mei X. Antioxidant activity of an exopolysaccharide purified from *Lactococcus lactis* subsp. lactis 12. Carbohydr Polym 2010; 80(3): 908-14.
[http://dx.doi.org/ 10.1016/j.carbpol.2010.01.005]

[369] Chen H, Zhang M, Qu Z, Xie B. Antioxidant activities of different fractions of polysaccharide conjugates from green tea (*Camellia Sinensis*). Food Chem 2008; 106(2): 559-63.
[http://dx.doi.org/ 10.1016/j.foodchem.2007.06.040]

[370] Jensen GS, Benson KF, Carter SG, Endres JR. GanedenBC30 cell wall and metabolites: anti-inflammatory and immune modulating effects *in vitro*. BMC Immunol 2010; 11(1): 15.
[http://dx.doi.org/ 10.1186/1471-2172-11-15] [PMID: 20331905]

[371] García-Carrizo F, Cannon B, Nedergaard J, *et al.* Regulation of thermogenic capacity in brown and white adipocytes by the prebiotic high-esterified pectin and its postbiotic acetate. Int J Obes 2020; 44(3): 715-26.
[http://dx.doi.org/ 10.1038/s41366-019-0445-6] [PMID: 31467421]

[372] Riaz Rajoka MS, Zhao H, Mehwish HM, *et al.* Anti-tumor potential of cell free culture supernatant of

Lactobacillus rhamnosus strains isolated from human breast milk. Food Res Int 2019; 123: 286-97. [http://dx.doi.org/ 10.1016/j.foodres.2019.05.002] [PMID: 31284979]

[373] Kalliomäki M, Salminen S, Arvilommi H, Kero P, Koskinen P, Isolauri E. Probiotics in primary prevention of atopic disease: a randomised placebo-controlled trial. Lancet 2001; 357(9262): 1076-9. [http://dx.doi.org/ 10.1016/S0140-6736(00)04259-8] [PMID: 11297958]

[374] Kim S-O, Ah Y-M, Yu YM, Choi KH, Shin W-G, Lee J-Y. Effects of probiotics for the treatment of atopic dermatitis: a meta-analysis of randomized controlled trials. Ann Allergy Asthma Immunol 2014; 113(2): 217-26. [http://dx.doi.org/ 10.1016/j.anai.2014.05.021] [PMID: 24954372]

[375] Salinas I, Díaz-Rosales P, Cuesta A, *et al.* Effect of heat-inactivated fish and non-fish derived probiotics on the innate immune parameters of a teleost fish (Sparus aurata L.). Vet Immunol Immunopathol 2006; 111(3-4): 279-86. [http://dx.doi.org/ 10.1016/j.vetimm.2006.01.020] [PMID: 16516307]

[376] Kawase M, He F, Miyazawa K, Kubota A, Yoda K, Hiramatsu M. Orally administered heat-killed *Lactobacillus gasseri* TMC0356 can upregulate cell-mediated immunity in senescence-accelerated mice. FEMS Microbiol Lett 2012; 326(2): 125-30. [http://dx.doi.org/ 10.1111/j.1574-6968.2011.02440.x] [PMID: 22092995]

[377] Maeda N, Nakamura R, Hirose Y, *et al.* Oral administration of heat-killed *Lactobacillus plantarum* L-137 enhances protection against influenza virus infection by stimulation of type I interferon production in mice. Int Immunopharmacol 2009; 9(9): 1122-5. [http://dx.doi.org/ 10.1016/j.intimp.2009.04.015] [PMID: 19410659]

[378] Goto H, Sagitani A, Ashida N, *et al.* Anti-influenza virus effects of both live and non-live *Lactobacillus acidophilus* L-92 accompanied by the activation of innate immunity. Br J Nutr 2013; 110(10): 1810-8. [http://dx.doi.org/ 10.1017/S0007114513001104] [PMID: 23594927]

[379] Fujii T, *et al.* Effects of heat-killed *Lactococcus lactis* subsp. lactis JCM 5805 on mucosal and systemic immune parameters, and antiviral reactions to influenza virus in healthy adults; a randomized controlled double-blind study. J Funct Foods 2017; 35: 513-21. [http://dx.doi.org/ 10.1016/j.jff.2017.06.011]

[380] Shigwedha N, Sichel L, Jia L, Al-Shura A N, Zhang L. Probiotics, paraprobiotics, and probiotical cell fragments (PCFs) as crisis management tools for important health problems 2020

[381] Taverniti V, Guglielmetti S. The immunomodulatory properties of probiotic microorganisms beyond their viability (ghost probiotics: proposal of paraprobiotic concept). Genes Nutr 2011; 6(3): 261-74. [http://dx.doi.org/ 10.1007/s12263-011-0218-x] [PMID: 21499799]

[382] Kanauchi O, Andoh A, AbuBakar S, Yamamoto N. Probiotics and paraprobiotics in viral infection: clinical application and effects on the innate and acquired immune systems. Curr Pharm Des 2018; 24(6): 710-7. [http://dx.doi.org/ 10.2174/1381612824666180116163411] [PMID: 29345577]

[383] Gerritsen J, Smidt H, Rijkers GT, de Vos WM. Intestinal microbiota in human health and disease: the impact of probiotics. Genes Nutr 2011; 6(3): 209-40. [http://dx.doi.org/ 10.1007/s12263-011-0229-7] [PMID: 21617937]

[384] Kimoto-Nira H, Mizumachi K, Okamoto T, Sasaki K, Kurisaki J. Influence of long-term consumption of a *Lactococcus lactis* strain on the intestinal immunity and intestinal flora of the senescence-accelerated mouse. Br J Nutr 2009; 102(2): 181-5. [http://dx.doi.org/ 10.1017/S0007114508143574] [PMID: 19586567]

[385] Ueno N, Fujiya M, Segawa S, *et al.* Heat-killed body of *Lactobacillus brevis* SBC8803 ameliorates intestinal injury in a murine model of colitis by enhancing the intestinal barrier function. Inflamm Bowel Dis 2011; 17(11): 2235-50. [http://dx.doi.org/ 10.1002/ibd.21597] [PMID: 21987297]

[386] Bermudez-Brito M, Plaza-Díaz J, Muñoz-Quezada S, Gómez-Llorente C, Gil A. Probiotic mechanisms of action. Ann Nutr Metab 2012; 61(2): 160-74.
[http://dx.doi.org/ 10.1159/000342079] [PMID: 23037511]

[387] Sun Z, Wang X, Andersson R. Role of intestinal permeability in monitoring mucosal barrier function. History, methodology, and significance of pathophysiology. Dig Surg 1998; 15(5): 386-97.
[http://dx.doi.org/ 10.1159/000018651] [PMID: 9845620]

[388] Generoso SV, Viana ML, Santos RG, *et al.* Protection against increased intestinal permeability and bacterial translocation induced by intestinal obstruction in mice treated with viable and heat-killed Saccharomyces boulardii. Eur J Nutr 2011; 50(4): 261-9.
[http://dx.doi.org/ 10.1007/s00394-010-0134-7] [PMID: 20936479]

[389] Zeng J, Jiang J, Zhu W, Chu Y. Heat-killed yogurt-containing lactic acid bacteria prevent cytokine-induced barrier disruption in human intestinal Caco-2 cells. Ann Microbiol 2016; 66(1): 171-8.
[http://dx.doi.org/ 10.1007/s13213-015-1093-2]

[390] Multicenter randomized controlled trial of heat killed *Lactobacillus acidophilus* LB in patients with chronic diarrhea. Chin J Dig Dis 2002; 3(4): 167-71.
[http://dx.doi.org/ 10.1046/j.1443-9573.2002.00095.x]

[391] Liévin-Le Moal V, Sarrazin-Davila LE, Servin AL. An experimental study and a randomized, double-blind, placebo-controlled clinical trial to evaluate the antisecretory activity of *Lactobacillus acidophilus* strain LB against nonrotavirus diarrhea. Pediatrics 2007; 120(4): e795-803.
[http://dx.doi.org/ 10.1542/peds.2006-2930] [PMID: 17768180]

[392] Tarrerias AL, Costil V, Vicari F, *et al.* The effect of inactivated Lactobacillus LB fermented culture medium on symptom severity: observational investigation in 297 patients with diarrhea-predominant irritable bowel syndrome. Dig Dis 2011; 29(6): 588-91.
[http://dx.doi.org/ 10.1159/000332987] [PMID: 22179215]

[393] Zheng B, van Bergenhenegouwen J, Overbeek S, *et al. Bifidobacterium* breve attenuates murine dextran sodium sulfate-induced colitis and increases regulatory T cell responses. PLoS One 2014; 9(5): e95441.
[http://dx.doi.org/ 10.1371/journal.pone.0095441] [PMID: 24787575]

[394] Imaoka A, Shima T, Kato K, *et al.* Anti-inflammatory activity of probiotic *Bifidobacterium*: enhancement of IL-10 production in peripheral blood mononuclear cells from ulcerative colitis patients and inhibition of IL-8 secretion in HT-29 cells. World J Gastroenterol 2008; 14(16): 2511-6.
[http://dx.doi.org/ 10.3748/wjg.14.2511] [PMID: 18442197]

[395] Shreiner AB, Kao JY, Young VB. The gut microbiome in health and in disease. Curr Opin Gastroenterol 2015; 31(1): 69-75.
[http://dx.doi.org/ 10.1097/MOG.0000000000000139] [PMID: 25394236]

[396] Homayouni-rad A, Fathi-zavoshti H, Douroud N, Shahbazi N, Abbasi A. Evaluating the Role of Postbiotics as a New Generation of Probiotics in Health and Diseases. J Ardabil Univ Med Sci 2020; 19(4): 381-99.
[http://dx.doi.org/ 10.29252/jarums.19.4.381]

[397] Ríos-Covián D, Ruas-Madiedo P, Margolles A, Gueimonde M, de Los Reyes-Gavilán CG, Salazar N. C. G. De Los Reyes-gavilán, and N. Salazar, "Intestinal short chain fatty acids and their link with diet and human health. Front Microbiol 2016; 7: 185.
[http://dx.doi.org/ 10.3389/fmicb.2016.00185] [PMID: 26925050]

[398] Louis P, Scott KP, Duncan SH, Flint HJ. Understanding the effects of diet on bacterial metabolism in the large intestine. J Appl Microbiol 2007; 102(5): 1197-208.
[http://dx.doi.org/ 10.1111/j.1365-2672.2007.03322.x] [PMID: 17448155]

[399] Rampengan NH, Manoppo J, Warouw SM. Comparison of efficacies between live and killed probiotics in children with lactose malabsorption. Southeast Asian J Trop Med Public Health 2010; 41(2): 474-81.

[PMID: 20578532]

[400] Oak SJ, Jha R. The effects of probiotics in lactose intolerance: A systematic review. Crit Rev Food Sci Nutr 2019; 59(11): 1675-83.
[http://dx.doi.org/ 10.1080/10408398.2018.1425977] [PMID: 29425071]

[401] Wegh , Carrie AM, Sharon Y, *et al.* Postbiotics and their potential applications in early life nutrition and beyond. Int J Mol Sci 2019; 20(19): 4673.
[http://dx.doi.org/ 10.3390/ijms20194673]

[402] Segawa S, Wakita Y, Hirata H, Watari J. Oral administration of heat-killed *Lactobacillus brevis* SBC8803 ameliorates alcoholic liver disease in ethanol-containing diet-fed C57BL/6N mice. Int J Food Microbiol 2008; 128(2): 371-7.
[http://dx.doi.org/ 10.1016/j.ijfoodmicro.2008.09.023] [PMID: 18976829]

[403] Wang Y, Liu Y, Sidhu A, Ma Z, McClain C, Feng W. *Lactobacillus rhamnosus* GG culture supernatant ameliorates acute alcohol-induced intestinal permeability and liver injury. Am J Physiol Gastrointest Liver Physiol 2012; 303(1): G32-41.
[http://dx.doi.org/ 10.1152/ajpgi.00024.2012] [PMID: 22538402]

[404] Li N, Russell WM, Douglas-escobar M, Hauser N, Lopez M, Neu J. Live and heat-killed *Lactobacillus rhamnosus* GG: effects on proinflammatory and anti-inflammatory cytokines/chemokines in gastrostomy-fed infant rats. Pediatr Res 2009; 66(2): 203-7.
[http://dx.doi.org/ 10.1203/PDR.0b013e3181aabd4f] [PMID: 19390478]

[405] Lopez M, Li N, Kataria J, Russell M, Neu J. Live and ultraviolet-inactivated *Lactobacillus rhamnosus* GG decrease flagellin-induced interleukin-8 production in Caco-2 cells. J Nutr 2008; 138(11): 2264-8.
[http://dx.doi.org/ 10.3945/jn.108.093658] [PMID: 18936229]

[406] Rafter J. The effects of probiotics on colon cancer development. Nutr Res Rev 2004; 17(2): 277-84.
[http://dx.doi.org/ 10.1079/NRR200484] [PMID: 19079931]

[407] Mansouri-Tehrani H-A, Rabbani-Khorasgani M, Hosseini S M, Mokarian F, Mahdavi H, Roayaei M. Effect of supplements: Probiotics and probiotic plus honey on blood cell counts and serum IgA in patients receiving pelvic radiotherapy Journal of research in medical sciences: the official journal of Isfahan University of Medical Sciences 2015; 20(7): 679.

[408] Österlund P, Ruotsalainen T, Korpela R, *et al. Lactobacillus* supplementation for diarrhoea related to chemotherapy of colorectal cancer: a randomised study. Br J Cancer 2007; 97(8): 1028-34.
[http://dx.doi.org/ 10.1038/sj.bjc.6603990] [PMID: 17895895]

[409] Tiptiri-Kourpeti A, Spyridopoulou K, Santarmaki V, *et al. Lactobacillus casei* exerts anti-proliferative effects accompanied by apoptotic cell death and up-regulation of TRAIL in colon carcinoma cells. PLoS One 2016; 11(2): e0147960.
[http://dx.doi.org/ 10.1371/journal.pone.0147960] [PMID: 26849051]

[410] Paparo L, Nocerino R, Di Scala C, *et al.* Targeting Food Allergy with Probiotics. Adv Exp Med Biol 2019; 1125: 57-68.
[http://dx.doi.org/ 10.1007/5584_2018_316] [PMID: 30680644]

[411] Gupta RS, Springston EE, Warrier MR, *et al.* The prevalence, severity, and distribution of childhood food allergy in the United States. Pediatrics 2011; 128(1): e9-e17.
[http://dx.doi.org/ 10.1542/peds.2011-0204] [PMID: 21690110]

[412] Prince BT, Mandel MJ, Nadeau K, Singh AM. Gut microbiome and the development of food allergy and allergic disease. Pediatr Clin North Am 2015; 62(6): 1479-92.
[http://dx.doi.org/ 10.1016/j.pcl.2015.07.007] [PMID: 26456445]

[413] Nowak-Węgrzyn A, Chatchatee P. Mechanisms of tolerance induction 2017.
[http://dx.doi.org/ 10.1159/000457915]

[414] Abbasi A, Hajipour N, Hasannezhad P, Baghbanzadeh A, Aghebati-Maleki L. Potential *in vivo* delivery routes of postbiotics. Crit Rev Food Sci Nutr 2020; 1-39.

[http://dx.doi.org/ 10.1080/10408398.2020.1865260] [PMID: 33356449]

[415] Noh DO, Kim SH, Gilliland SE. Incorporation of cholesterol into the cellular membrane of *Lactobacillus acidophilus* ATCC 43121. J Dairy Sci 1997; 80(12): 3107-13.
[http://dx.doi.org/ 10.3168/jds.S0022-0302(97)76281-7] [PMID: 9436091]

[416] Kimoto H, Ohmomo S, Okamoto T. Cholesterol removal from media by lactococci. J Dairy Sci 2002; 85(12): 3182-8.
[http://dx.doi.org/ 10.3168/jds.S0022-0302(02)74406-8] [PMID: 12512591]

[417] Iyadorai T, Mariappan V, Vellasamy KM, *et al.* Prevalence and association of pks+ Escherichia coli with colorectal cancer in patients at the University Malaya Medical Centre, Malaysia. PLoS One 2020; 15(1): e0228217.
[http://dx.doi.org/ 10.1371/journal.pone.0228217] [PMID: 31990962]

[418] Rad AH, Aghebati-Maleki L, Kafil HS, Abbasi A. Molecular mechanisms of postbiotics in colorectal cancer prevention and treatment. Crit Rev Food Sci Nutr 2020; 1-17.
[http://dx.doi.org/ 10.1080/10408398.2020.1765310] [PMID: 32410512]

[419] An BC, Ryu Y, Yoon YS, *et al.* Colorectal cancer therapy using a *Pediococcus pentosaceus* SL4 drug delivery system secreting lactic acid bacteria-derived protein p8. Mol Cells 2019; 42(11): 755-62.
[PMID: 31707776]

[420] da Costa R J, Voloski F L, Mondadori R G, Duval E H, Fiorentini Â M. Preservation of meat products with bacteriocins produced by lactic acid bacteria isolated from meat 2019.
[http://dx.doi.org/ 10.1155/2019/4726510]

[421] Foo H, Loh T, Abdul Mutalib N, Rahim R. The myth and therapeutic potentials of postbiotics. Microbiome and metabolome in diagnosis, therapy, and other strategic applications. Academic Press 2019; pp. 201-8.
[http://dx.doi.org/ 10.1016/B978-0-12-815249-2.00021-X]

[422] Johnson AC, Farmer AD, Ness TJ, Greenwood-Van Meerveld B. Critical evaluation of animal models of visceral pain for therapeutics development: A focus on irritable bowel syndrome. Neurogastroenterol Motil 2020; 32(4): e13776.
[http://dx.doi.org/ 10.1111/nmo.13776] [PMID: 31833625]

[423] Kamiya T, Wang L, Forsythe P, *et al.* Inhibitory effects of Lactobacillus reuteri on visceral pain induced by colorectal distension in Sprague-Dawley rats. Gut 2006; 55(2): 191-6.
[http://dx.doi.org/ 10.1136/gut.2005.070987] [PMID: 16361309]

[424] Shimizu K, Sato H, Suga Y, *et al.* The effects of *Lactobacillus pentosus* strain b240 and appropriate physical training on salivary secretory IgA levels in elderly adults with low physical fitness: a randomized, double-blind, placebo-controlled trial. J Clin Biochem Nutr 2014; 54(1): 61-6.
[http://dx.doi.org/ 10.3164/jcbn.13-62] [PMID: 24426193]

[425] Shinkai S, Toba M, Saito T, *et al.* Immunoprotective effects of oral intake of heat-killed *Lactobacillus pentosus* strain b240 in elderly adults: a randomised, double-blind, placebo-controlled trial. Br J Nutr 2013; 109(10): 1856-65.
[http://dx.doi.org/ 10.1017/S0007114512003753] [PMID: 22947249]

[426] Miyazawa K, Kawase M, Kubota A, *et al.* Heat-killed *Lactobacillus gasseri* can enhance immunity in the elderly in a double-blind, placebo-controlled clinical study. Benef Microbes 2015; 6(4): 441-9.
[http://dx.doi.org/ 10.3920/BM2014.0108] [PMID: 25653155]

[427] Kimoto-Nira H, Suzuki C, Kobayashi M, Sasaki K, Kurisaki J, Mizumachi K. Anti-ageing effect of a lactococcal strain: analysis using senescence-accelerated mice. Br J Nutr 2007; 98(6): 1178-86.
[http://dx.doi.org/ 10.1017/S0007114507787469] [PMID: 17617939]

[428] Burton JP, Drummond BK, Chilcott CN, *et al.* Influence of the probiotic *Streptococcus salivarius* strain M18 on indices of dental health in children: a randomized double-blind, placebo-controlled trial. J Med Microbiol 2013; 62(Pt 6): 875-84.

[http://dx.doi.org/ 10.1099/jmm.0.056663-0] [PMID: 23449874]

[429] Tanzer JM, Thompson A, Lang C, *et al.* Caries inhibition by and safety of *Lactobacillus paracasei* DSMZ16671. J Dent Res 2010; 89(9): 921-6.
[http://dx.doi.org/ 10.1177/0022034510369460] [PMID: 20519491]

[430] Saeki H, Furue M, Furukawa F, *et al.* Guidelines for management of atopic dermatitis. J Dermatol 2009; 36(10): 563-77.
[http://dx.doi.org/ 10.1111/j.1346-8138.2009.00706.x] [PMID: 19785716]

[431] Kang JS, Youm JK, Jeong SK, *et al.* Topical application of a novel ceramide derivative, K6PC-9, inhibits dust mite extract-induced atopic dermatitis-like skin lesions in NC/Nga mice. Int Immunopharmacol 2007; 7(13): 1589-97.
[http://dx.doi.org/ 10.1016/j.intimp.2007.08.009] [PMID: 17996668]

[432] Karki R, Jung M-A, Kim K-J, Kim D-W. Inhibitory effect of Nelumbo nucifera (Gaertn) on the development of atopic dermatitis-like skin lesions in NC/Nga mice. Evidence-Based Complementary and Alternative Medicine 2012; Vol. 2012.

[433] Kim JY, Park BK, Park HJ, Park YH, Kim BO, Pyo S. Atopic dermatitis-mitigating effects of new *Lactobacillus* strain, *Lactobacillus sakei* probio 65 isolated from Kimchi. J Appl Microbiol 2013; 115(2): 517-26.
[http://dx.doi.org/ 10.1111/jam.12229] [PMID: 23607518]

[434] Moroi M, Uchi S, Nakamura K, *et al.* Beneficial effect of a diet containing heat-killed *Lactobacillus paracasei* K71 on adult type atopic dermatitis. J Dermatol 2011; 38(2): 131-9.
[http://dx.doi.org/ 10.1111/j.1346-8138.2010.00939.x] [PMID: 21269308]

[435] Imperial IC, Ibana JA. Addressing the antibiotic resistance problem with probiotics: reducing the risk of its double-edged sword effect. Front Microbiol 2016; 7: 1983.
[http://dx.doi.org/ 10.3389/fmicb.2016.01983] [PMID: 28018315]

[436] Vijaya Kumar B, Vijayendra SVN, Reddy OVS. Trends in dairy and non-dairy probiotic products - a review. J Food Sci Technol 2015; 52(10): 6112-24.
[http://dx.doi.org/ 10.1007/s13197-015-1795-2] [PMID: 26396359]

[437] Weese JS, Martin H. Assessment of commercial probiotic bacterial contents and label accuracy. Can Vet J 2011; 52(1): 43-6.
[PMID: 21461205]

[438] Phister TG, O'Sullivan DJ, McKay LL. Identification of bacilysin, chlorotetaine, and iturin a produced by Bacillus sp. strain CS93 isolated from pozol, a Mexican fermented maize dough. Appl Environ Microbiol 2004; 70(1): 631-4.
[http://dx.doi.org/ 10.1128/AEM.70.1.631-634.2004] [PMID: 14711701]

[439] Palacios MC, Haros M, Sanz Y, Rosell CM. Selection of lactic acid bacteria with high phytate degrading activity for application in whole wheat breadmaking. Lebensm Wiss Technol 2008; 41(1): 82-92.
[http://dx.doi.org/ 10.1016/j.lwt.2007.02.005]

[440] Haros M, Bielecka M, Honke J, Sanz Y. Phytate-degrading activity in lactic acid bacteria. Pol J Food Nutr Sci 2008; 58(1)

[441] Shigwedha N. Probiotical cell fragments (PCFs) as "novel nutraceutical ingredients". J Biosci Med (Irvine) 2014; 2(03): 43.
[http://dx.doi.org/ 10.4236/jbm.2014.23007]

[442] Gabriele H. Requirements for a successful future of probiotics. Advances in probiotic technology. CRC Press 2015; pp. 147-53.
[http://dx.doi.org/ 10.1201/b18807-10]

[443] Shenderov BA, Sinitsa AV, Zakharchenko MM, Lang C. *METABIOTICS.* Present state, challenges and prerespectives. Springer, 2020.

[444] Klein G, Schanstra JP, Hoffmann J, Mischak H, Siwy J, Zimmermann K. Proteomics as a quality control tool of pharmaceutical probiotic bacterial lysate products. PLoS One 2013; 8(6): e66682.
[http://dx.doi.org/ 10.1371/journal.pone.0066682] [PMID: 23840518]

[445] Zihler A, Le Blay G, de Wouters T, *et al. In vitro* inhibition activity of different bacteriocin-producing Escherichia coli against Salmonella strains isolated from clinical cases. Lett Appl Microbiol 2009; 49(1): 31-8.
[http://dx.doi.org/ 10.1111/j.1472-765X.2009.02614.x] [PMID: 19413755]

[446] Konrad A, Mähler M, Flogerzi B, *et al.* Amelioration of murine colitis by feeding a solution of lysed Escherichia coli. Scand J Gastroenterol 2003; 38(2): 172-9.
[http://dx.doi.org/ 10.1080/00365520310000663] [PMID: 12678334]

[447] Przybilla B, Heppeler M, Ruzicka T. Preventive effect of an E. coli-filtrate (Colibiogen) in polymorphous light eruption. Br J Dermatol 1989; 121(2): 229-33.
[http://dx.doi.org/ 10.1111/j.1365-2133.1989.tb01803.x] [PMID: 2673324]

[448] Rudkowski Z, Bromirska J. Shortening of the period of fecal excretion of salmonella in infants under treatment with hylak forte. Padiatr Padol 1991; 26(2): 111-4.
[PMID: 1945464]

[449] Omarov T, Omarova L, Omarova V, Sarsenova S. The chronic gastritis, the dysbacteriosis and the use of Hylak forte at the treatment. 2014.

[450] Timko J. Probiotics as prevention of radiation-induced diarrhoea. J Radiother Pract 2010; 9(4): 201.
[http://dx.doi.org/ 10.1017/S1460396910000087]

[451] Ray S, Sherlock A, Wilken T, Woods T. Cell wall lysed probiotic tincture decreases immune response to pathogenic enteric bacteria and improves symptoms in autistic and immune compromised children. Explore (NY) 2010; 19(1): 1-5.
[PMID: 20129304]

[452] West R, Roberts E, Sichel L, Sichel J. Improvements in gastrointestinal symptoms among children with autism spectrum disorder receiving the Delpro® probiotic and immunomodulator formulation. J Prob Health 2013; 1(2)

[453] Kober M-M, Bowe WP. The effect of probiotics on immune regulation, acne, and photoaging. Int J Womens Dermatol 2015; 1(2): 85-9.
[http://dx.doi.org/ 10.1016/j.ijwd.2015.02.001] [PMID: 28491964]

[454] Callewaert C, Lambert J, Van de Wiele T. Towards a bacterial treatment for armpit malodour. Exp Dermatol 2017; 26(5): 388-91.
[http://dx.doi.org/ 10.1111/exd.13259] [PMID: 27892611]

[455] Probiotics-promising cosmetic ingredient or marketing tool? Personal Care, Cosmetics, Dermatology, Home Care and I 2016; I: 10.

[456] Holz C, Benning J, Schaudt M, *et al.* Novel bioactive from *Lactobacillus brevis* DSM17250 to stimulate the growth of Staphylococcus epidermidis: a pilot study. Benef Microbes 2017; 8(1): 121-31.
[http://dx.doi.org/ 10.3920/BM2016.0073] [PMID: 27824277]

[457] Pirozzi C, Lama A, Annunziata C, *et al.* Butyrate prevents valproate-induced liver injury: *In vitro* and *in vivo* evidence. FASEB J 2020; 34(1): 676-90.
[http://dx.doi.org/ 10.1096/fj.201900927RR] [PMID: 31914696]

[458] Rinaldi F, Trink A, Pinto D. Efficacy of postbiotics in a PRP-like cosmetic product for the treatment of alopecia area celsi: A randomized double-blinded parallel-group study. Dermatol Ther (Heidelb) 2020; 10(3): 483-93.
[http://dx.doi.org/ 10.1007/s13555-020-00369-9] [PMID: 32279227]

[459] Varian BJ, Poutahidis T, DiBenedictis BT, *et al.* Microbial lysate upregulates host oxytocin. Brain Behav Immun 2017; 61: 36-49.

[http://dx.doi.org/ 10.1016/j.bbi.2016.11.002] [PMID: 27825953]

[460] Swann JR, Spitzer SO, Diaz Heijtz R. Developmental signatures of microbiota-derived metabolites in the mouse brain. Metabolites 2020; 10(5): 172.
[http://dx.doi.org/ 10.3390/metabo10050172] [PMID: 32344839]

[461] Kareem KY, Loh TC, Foo HL, Akit H, Samsudin AA. Effects of dietary postbiotic and inulin on growth performance, IGF1 and GHR mRNA expression, faecal microbiota and volatile fatty acids in broilers. BMC Vet Res 2016; 12(1): 163.
[http://dx.doi.org/ 10.1186/s12917-016-0790-9] [PMID: 27496016]

[462] Choe DW, Loh TC, Foo HL, Hair-Bejo M, Awis QS. Egg production, faecal pH and microbial population, small intestine morphology, and plasma and yolk cholesterol in laying hens given liquid metabolites produced by *Lactobacillus plantarum* strains. Br Poult Sci 2012; 53(1): 106-15.
[http://dx.doi.org/ 10.1080/00071668.2012.659653] [PMID: 22404811]

[463] Kareem KY, Loh TC, Foo HL, Asmara SA, Akit H. Influence of postbiotic RG14 and inulin combination on cecal microbiota, organic acid concentration, and cytokine expression in broiler chickens. Poult Sci 2017; 96(4): 966-75.
[http://dx.doi.org/ 10.3382/ps/pew362] [PMID: 28339522]

[464] Loh TC, Choe DW, Foo HL, Sazili AQ, Bejo MH. Effects of feeding different postbiotic metabolite combinations produced by *Lactobacillus plantarum* strains on egg quality and production performance, faecal parameters and plasma cholesterol in laying hens. BMC Vet Res 2014; 10(1): 149.
[http://dx.doi.org/ 10.1186/1746-6148-10-149] [PMID: 24996258]

[465] Villamil L, Tafalla C, Figueras A, Novoa B. Evaluation of immunomodulatory effects of lactic acid bacteria in turbot (*Scophthalmus maximus*). Clin Diagn Lab Immunol 2002; 9(6): 1318-23.
[PMID: 12414767]

[466] Salinas I, Myklebust R, Esteban MA, Olsen RE, Meseguer J, Ringø E. *In vitro* studies of *Lactobacillus delbrueckii* subsp. lactis in Atlantic salmon (Salmo salar L.) foregut: tissue responses and evidence of protection against Aeromonas salmonicida subsp. salmonicida epithelial damage. Vet Microbiol 2008; 128(1-2): 167-77.
[http://dx.doi.org/ 10.1016/j.vetmic.2007.10.011] [PMID: 18054448]

[467] Sun Y-Z, Xia H-Q, Yang H-L, Wang Y-L, Zou W-C. TLR2 signaling may play a key role in the probiotic modulation of intestinal microbiota in grouper *Epinephelus coioides*. Aquaculture 2014; 430: 50-6.
[http://dx.doi.org/ 10.1016/j.aquaculture.2014.03.042]

[468] Lazado CC, Caipang CMA, Gallage S, Brinchmann MF, Kiron V. Expression profiles of genes associated with immune response and oxidative stress in Atlantic cod, Gadus morhua head kidney leukocytes modulated by live and heat-inactivated intestinal bacteria. Comp Biochem Physiol B Biochem Mol Biol 2010; 155(3): 249-55.
[http://dx.doi.org/ 10.1016/j.cbpb.2009.11.006] [PMID: 19931638]

[469] Dawood M A, Koshio S, Ishikawa M, Yokoyama S. Preservation of meat products with bacteriocins produced by lactic acid bacteria isolated from meat Journal of Food Quality 2019; 2019

[470] Singh ST, Kamilya D, Kheti B, Bordoloi B, Parhi J. Paraprobiotic preparation from Bacillus amyloliquefaciens FPTB16 modulates immune response and immune relevant gene expression in Catla catla (Hamilton, 1822). Fish Shellfish Immunol 2017; 66: 35-42.
[http://dx.doi.org/ 10.1016/j.fsi.2017.05.005] [PMID: 28476667]

[471] Boyd CE, Gross A. Use of probiotics for improving soil and water quality in aquaculture ponds. 1998.
[http://dx.doi.org/ 10.1007/978-1-4615-5407-3]

[472] Dawood MA, Koshio S, Ishikawa M, Yokoyama S. Effects of heat killed *Lactobacillus plantarum* (LP20) supplemental diets on growth performance, stress resistance and immune response of red sea bream, Pagrus major. Aquaculture 2015; 442: 29-36.
[http://dx.doi.org/ 10.1016/j.aquaculture.2015.02.005]

[473] Rodriguez-Estrada U, Satoh S, Haga Y, Fushimi H, Sweetman J. Effects of inactivated *Enterococcus faecalis* and mannan oligosaccharide and their combination on growth, immunity, and disease protection in rainbow trout. N Am J Aquaculture 2013; 75(3): 416-28.
[http://dx.doi.org/ 10.1080/15222055.2013.799620]

[474] Mohapatra S, Chakraborty T, Prusty A, Das P, Paniprasad K, Mohanta K. Use of different microbial probiotics in the diet of rohu, Labeo rohita fingerlings: effects on growth, nutrient digestibility and retention, digestive enzyme activities and intestinal microflora. Aquacult Nutr 2012; 18(1): 1-11.
[http://dx.doi.org/ 10.1111/j.1365-2095.2011.00866.x]

[475] Taoka Y, *et al.* Use of live and dead probiotic cells in tilapia *Oreochromis niloticus.* Fish Sci 2006; 72(4): 755-66.
[http://dx.doi.org/ 10.1111/j.1444-2906.2006.01215.x]

[476] Newaj-Fyzul A, Adesiyun AA, Mutani A, Ramsubhag A, Brunt J, Austin B. Bacillus subtilis AB1 controls Aeromonas infection in rainbow trout (Oncorhynchus mykiss, Walbaum). J Appl Microbiol 2007; 103(5): 1699-706.
[http://dx.doi.org/ 10.1111/j.1365-2672.2007.03402.x] [PMID: 17953580]

[477] LaPatra SE, Fehringer TR, Cain KD. A probiotic Enterobacter sp. provides significant protection against Flavobacterium psychrophilum in rainbow trout (Oncorhynchus mykiss) after injection by two different routes. Aquaculture 2014; 433: 361-6.
[http://dx.doi.org/ 10.1016/j.aquaculture.2014.06.022]

[478] Chaluvadi S, Hotchkiss AT, Yam K. Gut Microbiota: Impact of Probiotics, Prebiotics, Synbiotics, Pharmabiotics, and Postbiotics on Human Health. Probiotics, Prebiotics, and Synbiotics: Bioactive Foods in Health Promotion. Elsevier Inc. 2015; pp. 515-23.

[479] Jung M Y, Choi K C, Byung-Doo L, Min-Kyoung S, Boung-Jun O, Kim P I. Isolation and characterization of a proteinaceous antifungal compounds from Lactobacillus plantarum BC-K30 with probiotic properties. Korean society of biological engineering conference 2013; 216-6.

[480] Torino MI, Font de Valdez G, Mozzi F. Biopolymers from lactic acid bacteria. Novel applications in foods and beverages. Front Microbiol 2015; 6: 834.
[http://dx.doi.org/ 10.3389/fmicb.2015.00834] [PMID: 26441845]

[481] And HC, Hoover DG. Bacteriocins and their food applications. Compr Rev Food Sci Food Saf 2003; 2(3): 82-100.
[http://dx.doi.org/ 10.1111/j.1541-4337.2003.tb00016.x] [PMID: 33451234]

[482] Sola-Oladokun B, Culligan EP, Sleator RD. Engineered probiotics: applications and biological containment. Annu Rev Food Sci Technol 2017; 8: 353-70.
[http://dx.doi.org/ 10.1146/annurev-food-030216-030256] [PMID: 28125354]

[483] Amalaradjou MAR, Bhunia AK. Bioengineered probiotics, a strategic approach to control enteric infections. Bioengineered 2013; 4(6): 379-87.
[http://dx.doi.org/ 10.4161/bioe.23574] [PMID: 23327986]

[484] Yang G, Jiang Y, Yang W, *et al.* Effective treatment of hypertension by recombinant *Lactobacillus plantarum* expressing angiotensin converting enzyme inhibitory peptide. Microb Cell Fact 2015; 14(1): 202.
[http://dx.doi.org/ 10.1186/s12934-015-0394-2] [PMID: 26691527]

[485] Zhang B, Li A, Zuo F, *et al.* Recombinant *Lactococcus lactis* NZ9000 secretes a bioactive kisspeptin that inhibits proliferation and migration of human colon carcinoma HT-29 cells. Microb Cell Fact 2016; 15(1): 102.
[http://dx.doi.org/ 10.1186/s12934-016-0506-7] [PMID: 27287327]

[486] Ma Y, Liu J, Hou J, *et al.* Oral administration of recombinant *Lactococcus lactis* expressing HSP65 and tandemly repeated P277 reduces the incidence of type I diabetes in non-obese diabetic mice. PLoS One 2014; 9(8): e105701.

[http://dx.doi.org/ 10.1371/journal.pone.0105701] [PMID: 25157497]

[487] Robert S, Gysemans C, Takiishi T, *et al.* Oral delivery of glutamic acid decarboxylase (GAD)-65 and IL10 by *Lactococcus lactis* reverses diabetes in recent-onset NOD mice. Diabetes 2014; 63(8): 2876-87.
[http://dx.doi.org/ 10.2337/db13-1236] [PMID: 24677716]

[488] Villaño D, Gironés-Vilapana A, García-Viguera C, Moreno D. Development of functional foods. Innovation Strategies in the Food Industry. Elsevier 2016; pp. 191-210.
[http://dx.doi.org/ 10.1016/B978-0-12-803751-5.00010-6]

[489] Charoensiddhi S, Lorbeer AJ, Franco CM, Su P, Conlon MA, Zhang W. Process and economic feasibility for the production of functional food from the brown alga Ecklonia radiata. Algal Res 2018; 29: 80-91.
[http://dx.doi.org/ 10.1016/j.algal.2017.11.022]

[490] Shafipour Yordshahi A, Moradi M, Tajik H, Molaei R. Design and preparation of antimicrobial meat wrapping nanopaper with bacterial cellulose and postbiotics of lactic acid bacteria. Int J Food Microbiol 2020; 321: 108561.
[http://dx.doi.org/ 10.1016/j.ijfoodmicro.2020.108561] [PMID: 32078868]

[491] Barros CP, *et al.* Paraprobiotics, postbiotics and psychobiotics: concepts and potential applications in dairy products. Curr Opin Food Sci 2019.

[492] Taheri A, Jafari SM. Gum-based nanocarriers for the protection and delivery of food bioactive compounds. Adv Colloid Interface Sci 2019; 269: 277-95.
[http://dx.doi.org/ 10.1016/j.cis.2019.04.009] [PMID: 31132673]

[493] Homayoni Rad A, Vaghef Mehrabany E, Alipoor B, Vaghef Mehrabany L. The comparison of food and supplement as probiotic delivery vehicles. Crit Rev Food Sci Nutr 2016; 56(6): 896-909.
[http://dx.doi.org/ 10.1080/10408398.2012.733894] [PMID: 25117939]

[494] Oehlke K, Adamiuk M, Behsnilian D, *et al.* Potential bioavailability enhancement of bioactive compounds using food-grade engineered nanomaterials: a review of the existing evidence. Food Funct 2014; 5(7): 1341-59.
[http://dx.doi.org/ 10.1039/c3fo60067j] [PMID: 24752749]

[495] Ting Y, Jiang Y, Ho C-T, Huang Q. Common delivery systems for enhancing *in vivo* bioavailability and biological efficacy of nutraceuticals. J Funct Foods 2014; 7: 112-28.
[http://dx.doi.org/ 10.1016/j.jff.2013.12.010]

[496] de Vos P, Faas MM, Spasojevic M, Sikkema J. Encapsulation for preservation of functionality and targeted delivery of bioactive food components. Int Dairy J 2010; 20(4): 292-302.
[http://dx.doi.org/ 10.1016/j.idairyj.2009.11.008]

[497] Badea G, Lăcătuşu I, Badea N, Ott C, Meghea A. Use of various vegetable oils in designing photoprotective nanostructured formulations for UV protection and antioxidant activity. Ind Crops Prod 2015; 67: 18-24.
[http://dx.doi.org/ 10.1016/j.indcrop.2014.12.049]

[498] Shimoni E. Nanotechnology for foods: delivery systems. Global issues in food science and technology. Elsevier 2009; pp. 411-24.
[http://dx.doi.org/ 10.1016/B978-0-12-374124-0.00023-5]

[499] Liu J, Hu W, Chen H, Ni Q, Xu H, Yang X. Isotretinoin-loaded solid lipid nanoparticles with skin targeting for topical delivery. Int J Pharm 2007; 328(2): 191-5.
[http://dx.doi.org/ 10.1016/j.ijpharm.2006.08.007] [PMID: 16978810]

[500] Tamjidi F, Shahedi M, Varshosaz J, Nasirpour A. Nanostructured lipid carriers (NLC): A potential delivery system for bioactive food molecules. Innov Food Sci Emerg Technol 2013; 19: 29-43.
[http://dx.doi.org/ 10.1016/j.ifset.2013.03.002]

www.ingramcontent.com/pod-product-compliance
Lightning Source LLC
Chambersburg PA
CBHW041716210326
41598CB00007B/673